Understanding Cancer

Understanding Cancer

*An Invaluable Book for
Cancer Patients and Their Families*

MARILYN DUNLOP
**With a Preface by
RICHARD HASSELBACK, B.A., M.D., F.R.C.P.(C)**

Irwin Publishing
TORONTO CANADA

Copyright © 1985 Marilyn Dunlop
Preface Copyright © 1985 Richard Hasselback

Canadian Cataloguing in Publication Data

Dunlop, Marilyn, 1928-
  Understanding cancer

ISBN 0-7725-1507-7

1. Cancer. 2. Cancer — Psychological aspects.
I. Title.

RC263.D85 1985   616.99'4   C84-099028-6

Designed by Lisa Guthro for Robert Garbutt Productions
Typeset by ART-U Graphics Ltd.
Printed in Canada by Webcom Limited

1 2 3 4 5 6 7 8 WC 92 91 90 89 88 87 86 85

Published by Irwin Publishing Inc.

Contents

Preface

In the past quarter century cancer has become a subject people can discuss openly. It is no longer a socially unacceptable topic. Cancers are not rare diseases—29% of us will develop some type of cancer in our lifetime and one in five of us will die of a cancer at present rates. More than half of all families will be affected by cancer.

Yet a generation ago, the individual or family affected by a cancer would be fearful of the stigma that could result if acquaintances or fellow workers found out about a cancer in the family. This secrecy was not extended to heart disease, or even infectious diseases such as tuberculosis. Certainly there were and are grounds for fearing cancer because many individuals affected will eventually die of the disease. There were some who thought of it as an "unclean disease" that had to be hidden away and some people had the misconception that cancer was infectious or contagious. It is to be hoped misconceptions such as these, which, in themselves, do great harm to cancer patients, are disappearing. Relatively few people today think of a diagnosis of cancer in themselves or family members as something to be ashamed of. It can now be revealed and discussed.

And this is an important step. Open discussion about cancer is necessary if people are to cope with the disease. When a cancer develops in a family member, we regularly see the patient and family trying to become informed and understand the disease which has effects on all members of the family.

The danger exists today that in such discussions, misunderstandings, inaccuracies, fallacies, and errors are perpetuated and spread through the community. Only when sources of accurate reliable information about cancer in words intelligible to the non-professional are available to the public can the true facts be made known to those willing and anxious to becomed educated about this family of diseases.

We should be talking of "cancers" rather than just the singular "cancer." For cancers are a whole group of diseases just as infections are a group of diseases. We can no more think of cancers as different as skin cancer, acute leukemia, or cancers of the breast or lung as one disease than we can group together the many different kinds of infections such as the common cold, tuberculosis, typhoid fever, or malaria, all infectious diseases which affect human beings. Each type of cancer has its own causative factors, symptoms, signs, treatment and prognosis. The major underlying differences between these various cancers is in the organ or tissue in which they arise. That is the most important factor which determines the behaviour of the disease and the outlook for the patient.

But cancers do have some features in common. All are disorders of growth. None are infectious and only a few rare kinds are truly hereditary. Most are probably caused, or at least stimulated, by factors in our environment, different factors for different cancers.

Most cancers are chronic diseases: that is, they are illnesses of relatively slow onset and the course of the illness usually lasts over a period of months or years. Even when cured, the emotional and social consequences of a diagnosis of cancer can last a lifetime. Because of this, cancers have great psychological as well as physical effects on not only the patient, but on the family, friends, and co-workers as well. Understanding the stress created by a diagnosis of cancer on all concerned is necessary if those who make up the social environment of the cancer patient are going to be able to cope with those stresses.

Because cancer is a chronic disease, serious financial problems may arise. These will be most severe when the patient with cancer is the principal family provider, but even when others are affected, the expenses can be substantial for such items as drugs and transportation.

Because of our virtually universal health care insurance scheme, Canadians as individuals rarely face the massive medical expenses which can affect residents of other countries for items such as hospitalization, surgery, radiotherapy, and the cost of complex chemotherapeutic agents. Not only are Canadians provided with excellent facilities for the treatment of cancer but the cost of such care is spread evenly through the community as a whole and not imposed exclusively on the individuals who have the misfortune to have the cancer and require the use of those facilities. Cancer surgery is available in many primary care community hospitals. Radiotherapy equipment and the radiation oncology specialists trained to use it are generally concentrated in larger centres but widely distributed in Canada. Cancer chemotherapy drugs are available in many hospitals and the medical oncologists trained in the use of these drugs and overall management of cancer patients are becoming available in more of the smaller Canadian cities.

The overall facilities in Canada for the management of cancer are equal to any in the world and superior to those in many countries. Furthermore, efforts to improve both our understanding of cancer and our ability to treat it are a central ongoing objective of all Canadian cancer specialists.

Canada has had many pioneers in the study of the understanding and treatment of cancer. Dr. M. Vera Peters of Toronto was the first physician to recognize that Hodgkin's disease, once considered inevitably fatal, was a curable cancer. The cobalt radiotherapy unit which is still widely used throughout the world for the administration of radiotherapy was developed in Saskatoon and in Chalk River, Ontario by Dr. Harold Johns and co-workers. Dr. Robert Noble, then of London and more recently of Vancouver, discovered the periwinkle family of drugs which are mainstays in cancer chemotherapy. Dr. Mary Vachon is one of the world pioneers in exploring the emotional stresses cancer imposes not only on patients and their families but on the health team caring for the patients. In basic research, Drs. E. A. McCulloch and James Till developed techniques which permit an understanding of the fundamental derangement of growth that underlies certain cancers and Drs. Robert Bruce and Emmanuel Farber of Toronto and Dr. Hans Stich of Vancouver have explored causative factors of cancer and, by implication, ways that the incidence of cancer could be decreased.

Much of the support for such cancer research in Canada, and a great deal of public education and personal assistance to cancer patients is provided by the efforts of the Canadian Cancer Society, a group of lay volunteers who give freely of their time. There are few volunteer organizations in the world comparable to the Canadian Cancer Society in their dedication to a cause.

In this excellent book, Marilyn Dunlop makes available to patients and families information and insight that will help them to deal with an illness. Ignorance increases fear. Families facing a diagnosis of cancer will be better prepared to discuss their problems amongst themselves and with their health care team when a basic understanding of what they face is available to them.

RICHARD HASSELBACK, B.A., M.D., F.R.C.P.(C)
October, 1984

Understanding Cancer

Introduction

WHEN CANCER IS diagnosed, patients and those closest to them suddenly find themselves in unfamiliar territory. A multitude of questions tumble through their minds.

As a medical reporter for a large newspaper for more than fifteen years, I've received calls and letters from hundreds of people seeking sources of information about cancer. Possibly the most common query is whether I know of a book that would help them understand what is happening to them, that would explain treatment and assist in translating strange new words they're hearing.

I consider a request for information a good sign. It indicates a patient wants to be well enough informed to be able to ask intelligent questions of the doctors and actively take part, with cancer specialists, in the battle against his or her disease. It may mean family members or intimate friends want to know how to help a patient in practical day-to-day ways and provide emotional support.

This book has been put together with the help of patients and former patients who know from their own experience what information proved useful to them in their duels with the disease.

Volunteers and health professionals on the front line and experts from the Canadian Cancer Society and the National Cancer Institute of Canada also provided invaluable assistance.

Doctors treating the patient are, of course, the best source of information. Because each person is unique, each case is different. There are no pat answers that apply to everybody.

The primary aim of this book is to help lighten two burdens that commonly accompany cancer: fear of the unknown and a sense of helplessness.

We fear most the things we don't comprehend. Some fear is needless. It may stem from misinformation. In some instances friends who had cancer at a time when treatments available today did not exist may give the patient out-dated views, arising from their own experiences. In other cases, people with a kind of cancer that is commonly treated successfully may believe that all cancer is an inevitable threat to life. Understanding cancer may rid you of groundless fears.

To overcome feelings of helplessness is to refuse to let cancer attack the spirit. Science is only scratching the surface in understanding how the mind and body interact to combat disease. But there is no doubt that to feel beaten and unable to help yourself can't enhance health.

My hope is that as you make the journey through this segment of your life, this book will be a helpful guide.

MARILYN DUNLOP

PART ONE
The Personal Side of Cancer

One
The emotional impact

A WISE AND humane cancer specialist, Dr. Vera Peters of Toronto, addressing colleagues on the day she retired after many years of treating patients, gave them an important message. The emotional voyage for people with cancer can be far more painful than the physical one, she said.

Cancer ignites an emotional reaction like no other disease. Other diseases may be more disabling, more life-threatening than cancer, yet instilled in our society is the myth that cancer means pain and death.

No matter how many people you know who are well and busy, even though they were treated for cancer years earlier, your gut reaction when cancer is diagnosed is likely to be "Dear God, I am going to die."

You may be quite wrong. You may not die of cancer at all. You may outlive your whole family, dying in your sleep at the age of 95. What is ahead for you may not be dying of cancer but learning to live with it. It will be a challenge.

As many people who live with cancer have found, the blinkers are off. Never again will you hold the conviction you are invincible and fully in control of your own destiny. It is, in a sense, a loss of childish innocence.

Yet there do seem to be some landmarks on the voyage. A number of patients, looking back over the route they travelled, say they recall distinct stages. There were times, they say, when it might have helped them to know that others had similar experiences and had emerged intact emotionally.

For some, the first leg was the worst and it began when they were first told they had cancer.

At that stage, a patient may flatly refuse to believe the diagnosis. The mind won't accept it. It twists and turns, arguing, denying, blanking out or whirling away to trivial thoughts. "I'm too well to have cancer," one patient told himself. "Cancer is something other people get. The guy down the street, not me. The doctor is wrong."

Although people vary enormously in how they feel when the news is broken, it is not unusual to feel as if your brain is a caged animal, scurrying around and around in futile frenzy. It won't let you sleep. Food is hard to choke down. Concentration is impossible. "I had to hang on tight to keep from flying apart," said one man.

Doctors say it commonly takes several days before the emotional turmoil begins to subside and the person can think rationally about treatment and discuss it realistically. But, say the doctors, it is impressive to see how resilient cancer patients can be as they come to terms with the reality of cancer. Many find strength and courage they didn't know was in them.

To be keenly aware of your own mortality is an unfamiliar sensation. As one woman put it, "I came to see it as living with an unpredictable lion. It frightened other people and it scared me too. It appeared tame today but we knew it could turn on me anytime. For quite a long time I was so terrified of being mauled tomorrow, I lost sight of my todays."

Until about ten years ago, health professionals paid little heed to the emotional side of cancer. The focus of research and treatment was entirely on saving lives. Time and thought was not put into discovering how to relieve psychological pain. Patients and people who love them muddled through their own distresses as best they could. Some families collapsed in emotional ruins.

But as the number of people living with cancer increased, it became apparent there was more to cancer care than medical treatment. Patients themselves were among the first to realise it and do something about helping each other cope. Self-help groups began popping up. One of the first was Reach to

Recovery, for women with breast cancer, begun in 1952 by a New York woman, Terese Lasser. At the time, cancer patients were discouraged from discussing their treatment with each other, but Mrs. Lasser, who had had a mastectomy (removal of a breast or breasts), believed a woman who had made the psychological adjustment to the surgery could help new patients. About the same time, other cancer patients in the U.S. formed the Cured Cancer Club, a forerunner of today's Coping with Cancer programmes.

In the last decade there has been an explosion of research into the psychological and human side of cancer. It has been recognized that the health of a patient's spirit is equally as important as the health of the patient's body. From these studies and the experiences of patients much has been learned that may, to some measure, smooth the path for others. Each patient and family has their own special strengths and weaknesses and there is no one right way of coping with cancer suited to all. Furthermore, for every patient and the surrounding circle of people, the impact of cancer, like a kaleidoscope, is ever changing.

Some people continue to deny they have cancer. You wouldn't likely be reading this book if you are pretending to yourself cancer couldn't happen to you. But you may be anxious about a patient who is doing so, fearing they've lost contact with reality.

Don't be alarmed. There is nothing abnormal about taking time to face up to cancer. We have built-in mechanisms that protect us by blocking out shocks that would be too great to absorb in a single impact. They're like dams that hold back an overpowering rush of awareness. They let it seep in gradually. As long as it does not interfere with the patient's willingness to have treatment, there is no need to force recognition of cancer. For certain people, denying cancer is the best protection they can muster against unbearable anxiety. A number of them persuade themselves the treatment prescribed is merely "preventive." That's fine. In any case, no amount of information will convince a person who really needs to deny the facts.

One mother was upset when her teen-age son scoffed at the idea he had cancer despite the treatment he was undergoing. She thought by denying the nature of his disease he was not going to put up a strong fight against it. Yet he was using denial as a form of hope that he'd be with his buddies on the ski slopes before too long. It was spurring him to co-operate in every way he could with his doctors. Had he admitted to having cancer, he might have despaired of ever again flying over snow hills with his friends. His zest for life might have shrivelled.

Sensitive doctors may tell a patient the diagnosis in a gradual way so the shock isn't abrupt when the final word from diagnostic tests comes in. But not every patient is fortunate enough to have gentle handling. Even when they do, it is a hard blow.

Sometimes doctors ask family members to come with patients to appointments when the news is to be broken and it is useful to have a second pair of ears hear accurately what the doctor says. Doctors know, at this time, a patient may not be able to take in much information. The shock is too great.

A patient, however, may choose to see the doctor alone or may hear the diagnosis by phone. A few people stoically decide to keep the diagnosis secret. They ask their doctors not to tell family members. Patients who have tried that say it is a mistake. "Cancer can be unutterably lonely. No one should try to bear it alone," one person said. "If it isn't revealed, family and friends are robbed of the opportunity to share feelings and anxieties that arise."

Sooner or later, those closest to the patient find out. Hiding cancer is impossible. Their distress and worry about the future, both for the patient and for themselves, is often as great as the patient's. It's not uncommon for a patient to feel guilt for causing loved ones to suffer, illogical as such guilt may be.

Most difficult is telling children when a parent has cancer. Yet even young children rapidly pick up silent signals that something is wrong. Trying to spare them may only make them more distressed. They may imagine the situation to be worse than it really is, or believe it is their fault. Feeling shut out is harder for a child than knowing a parent is ill.

How the disease is explained, of course, depends on the age of the child. But child psychologists say parents should not wait until the child asks for an explanation. A child who asks no questions is not unaware something is wrong, but is too anxious to ask. It must be so terrible that it can't be talked about, the child may fear. Studies have shown that children who are not told can become depressed and withdrawn or may act rebelliously, developing behaviour problems and adding to family difficulties. It is their way of dealing with feelings of hurt they don't understand.

Family members, like patients, often need time to let the reality of the diagnosis sink in. For a while, the family may be out of step emotionally. One person may come to grips with cancer and want to talk about it before others are ready. There is a potential for conflict at the very time family members need each other most.

In some families, people are able to discuss cancer with everybody but the patient, in effect putting outside the circle of support the person they are trying to protect. In others, people become so solicitous they hover like mother hens until the patient wants to scream "Get off my back. Let me forget for a moment."

Sometimes a patient can feel rejected, over-protected and misunderstood all at the same time.

What is to be done? It is important to let the patient call the shots, indicating when he or she wants to talk openly about feelings.

In families that customarily talk over anything and everything, it may be only a matter of being sensitive enough to avoid pushing the sharing of feelings before the patient is ready. In others, in which people are accustomed to keeping emotions inside, it may be more difficult to express themselves openly in ways that help ease the awful loneliness of cancer.

Sometimes the patient would like to talk about it but doesn't know how to begin, afraid it will be too upsetting to the others. In other cases, the family may be so intent on keeping up the patient's spirits they present a front of determined cheerfulness that allows no opportunity for the patient to admit to fear and depression.

Watch for signals the patient wants to let out anxiety by talking with you. If you're looking for them, you will notice clues. Arrange opportunities for quiet conversation. Let the patient take the lead or ask if it is time to share feelings, rather than barging in. If the patient does want to talk, listen. Don't override with false optimism expressions of fear and anxiety. It is not going to convince the patient everything is fine and he or she will probably conclude you simply don't understand. On the other hand, if the patient is failing to see genuine reasons for optimism, it may help to provide a gentle reminder that they exist.

Some patients don't want to share their cancer battle with family. They want home to be their refuge from the struggle, where cancer isn't mentioned and life goes on as normally as ever.

If the patient is the most important person in the world to you, that may not be easy. Cancer is affecting *your* life intensely too. It's natural to worry about your own future as well as the patient's. One wife said, "My husband would say 'It's my cancer. Let me deal with it myself.' He didn't like me letting him know I was upset. But it wasn't just his life that his cancer was going to affect. It was mine too."

The wife of another patient said she felt guilty and selfish. "There I was thinking 'What's going to happen to me?' when all my concern should have been for Harry."

Cancer often forces major adjustments in families and it is easier on everybody if the necessary changes can be talked about and planned with the patient. But if the patient flatly refuses, all you can do is try to understand that the patient cannot accept the idea of change.

Patients may sense relatives drawing away from them emotionally. Unconsciously, the relatives may be reacting to the myth that cancer means death and be preparing themselves for the loss. They don't intentionally send out the message that they no longer want to be close to the patient, yet that is what it may appear to be and the patient feels isolated, hurt and confused.

If you are a person a patient looks to for emotional support, you need great insight into your own feelings. If you can hold up to the light and examine your built-in views of cancer, you may be able to see if you are grieving prematurely and be able to overcome it so you don't unwittingly withdraw, leaving your patient mired in loneliness.

Touch can overcome a patient's sense of alienation like nothing else. Hugging and stroking are powerful antidotes to the devastating feelings of being contaminated and unaccepted. It isn't uncommon to hear patients say they feel as if they are treated as modern-day lepers.

Nurses who have taken special training in the healing power of touch have observed how frequently it brings patients comfort of mind as well as body. "Giving back rubs may do much more than we used to realize," says one nurse. Patients have said a simple gesture of touch, having their hand held or a pat on the back, has felt enormously reassuring.

The wife of one patient said she had moved into the spare bedroom, thinking her husband would sleep better alone, until she realized how much he wanted her physical closeness each night. "The touch of my body next to his seemed to be soothing," she said.

Specialists in cancer psychology extol the value of touch and physical closeness. Nevertheless you can only do what is comfortable for you. The last thing a patient needs, when cancer has already forced many changes, is for you to change too and try to be somebody you are not.

If you are the patient, this tumultuous stage during which you and those around you are adjusting to the idea of cancer may test you sorely. Home may seem like anything but a haven.

You may feel nobody in the family knows what you are going through and those you look to most for support aren't giving it. When your own needs are so great, it is hard to realize that those you love are also dealing with their own tangled skeins of feelings.

You may be able to accept your disease before they can. You should be the one who sets the pattern for how openly you want cancer to be discussed in your home. But it may not be easy to speak out for yourself at a time when you are emotionally shaky.

If an unwanted discussion is being forced on you, you can say "I can't talk about it yet, although I know you are trying to help." Maybe you find it tricky to let others know your wishes without making them feel you are rejecting their help. But a pat on the arm with your words can take away any sting.

You may feel irritated about being required to handle your family with kid gloves right now. Yet, if you stop to think about it, you know it can be more painful to accept illness in people dearest to you than in yourself.

Possibly you need to vent the anger you feel about what has happened to you or you want to talk about your fears but you find you can't get through to those closest to you. "My husband just won't believe I have cancer," said one young woman. "He says I eat as much as he does. I look the same as always and I haven't any pain, so how could I have a tumour? He won't discuss it at all." She added sadly, "It's shut a door between us. My friend says he loves me too much to be able to accept my cancer. I like to think she's right. But I still wonder if we'll ever be as close again as we were before."

Another patient, speaking of her husband and daughter, said "I have to be *their* strength."

If your family is unable to provide emotional help, you may have to turn to a friend to be your sounding board and outlet for pent-up feelings. Sometimes only another person with cancer knows well enough what you are experiencing to make it easy for you to talk. A visiting volunteer or a patient group may prove indispensable. Many cancer treatment centres have patient groups or your doctor or local cancer society may be able to put you in touch with a volunteer visiting programme.

Maybe your family is overly-protective, so frightened for you they wrap you in a cocoon. You wish they'd back off. You can ask if they'll agree to a deal. "If you'll treat me the same as you did before my diagnosis," you say, "I promise that when I need your concern I'll ask for it." Then do it, otherwise a day may come when you feel you've been abandoned and you'll be full of self pity.

What makes cancer so hard to adjust to is its uncertainty. "Uncertainty is cancer's middle name," says one man. "It throws a monkey wrench into your future."

How a patient reacts to that uncertainty often depends on the stage of life as well as on personality. The young patient may need to lash out in anger. The hostility is to the situation, not the family, although they catch the brunt of the rage. Young people are, typically, geared to the future and cancer cannot help but seem dreadfully unfair. What will it do to their plans for a career, to their dreams of love and marriage? What will it do to their looks and to their sexuality? The threat of so many losses is brutal. Small wonder they are often consumed with fury.

People in their senior years are more likely to feel depressed. They don't want to be a burden on others and they may imagine the grim prospect of loss of independence and of the ability to look after themselves.

Those in mid-life are often already facing heavy demands on their emotional capacities as they adjust to their children growing up and leaving home, careers peaking, physical appearance changing with age, and the deaths of their own parents. The added stress of cancer may seem overwhelming.

A patient you love, however, may not fit the age pattern that is most typical. A young person may show an astonishing degree of maturity and face his disease with equanimity. A grandfather, who has been a fists-up fighter all his life, may come out swinging, ready to do battle.

Nobody can really tell you how you are going to react to cancer. But, in general, patients agree they have had one experience in common. No matter how good the outlook of treatment may be, they say, death seems closer than it ever did before.

You may feel nothing will ever be the same again. You are right. But that doesn't mean the change will be all for the worse. There are hundreds of people living with cancer today, who would tell you they might never have known how rich life can be had it not been for their tumours. Cancer opened their eyes and their hearts. Families have found warmth and closeness. Love has been shown and spoken that had long been submerged in the hurly-burly of daily routines. Beauty has become visible.

"We'd probably never have got to know Dad," said the 20-year-old son of a high-powered lawyer. "Until he got cancer he was working day and night. He'd have dropped dead of a heart attack if he'd kept that up. But the last couple of years we've had some great times together. He says it took the big C to get his priorities right."

"My wife is quite a bit younger than I am and I guess I had always treated her as a child," said a 55-year-old patient." She sure surprised me. She's given mie strength. I never realized how good the love of a mature woman would be."

It may be tough to see how any good can come out of your cancer. All you want to do is be rid of it.

There is something you can do right now. You can hope.

"When I had heart surgery a few years ago, friends sent me funny or naughty cards," says one man. "When I went to hospital for cancer surgery, they sent cards that said 'We're praying for you'. The message this time was 'You're not going to make it'."

With negative signals from many directions, it can be hard to sustain hope. But studies with patients have shown that it is precisely in situations of apparent helplessness that we most need the ability to hope. It is the one way of coping we have left. And it can have a powerful influence against stress.

In an educational book for health professionals prepared by the U.S. Department of Health and Human Resources, there is a quote from a physician, written in 1789. It says: "The desire for life is a very powerful stimulus in prolonging it, especially when that desire is supported by hope.... Despair of recovery is the beginning of death in all diseases."

Hope has been defined as confidence in survival. It is the opposite of giving up. Nobody can tell you how long you will live, so it isn't false hope to feel optimistic you will live for a long time.

If the statistics for your kind of cancer show, for example, that 70 per cent of patients are free of disease after five years, hope encourages you to put yourself among the winners. Hope lets you believe the outcome of treatment will justify any discomfort you might experience by undergoing it.

Doctors sometimes shy away from hope because they know unscrupulous con artists play on hope ruthlessly in order to sell their useless products. They have also seen patients work themselves into false euphoric hopefulness to the point where they refuse treatment that could have saved their lives. Such people have become so supremely confident of magic, spontaneous cures, they perceive no need for treatment. That kind of extreme unrealistic hope can be tragic.

But, at the other extreme, a person devoid of hope may also refuse treatment, convinced death is inevitable no matter what is done.

Hope is volatile in some people. Each slight change sends their hopes up or down dramatically. They need a lot of reassurance and may put their families through emotional wringers. Outside professional help may be required in extreme cases that teeter on the brink of mental illness.

The majority of patients, however, settle into a state of hope based on reality. It doesn't wipe out all the down days, but at times when distress surfaces they are aware their spirits will rise again. Hope gives patients the energy and the motivation to take an active part, with their doctors and families, in the attempt to defeat their diseases.

While it is cruel to patients to raise false hopes, we all need to believe that progress against cancer is being made. If cancer scientists maintained no hope, there would be no research. Without public hope, cancer research would not be financially supported and millions of people wouldn't be living reasonably normal lives with cancer today.

Hope is an important ingredient of your spirit. "It turns you around," says one cancer veteran, "It makes you say to yourself 'At the moment of diagnosis I was not from then on dying. I was living with this disease. I don't know how long I'll live. I didn't know before I got cancer how long I'd live. But right now I have cancer and I'm convinced I am going to live."

Just what is this disease you are going to live with? In the next chapter we will examine cancer, its whys and wherefores.

Two
The changing picture of cancer

SINCE THE EARLIEST written records of medicine were made 3,500 years ago, cancer has been observed in people and in animals. Yet only in our lifetime has there been any real progress in saving lives of those who develop it.

In our grandparents' generation the word "cancer" was usually spoken only in whispers, out of earshot of patients or children. It was simply too terrifying, too devoid of hope, to be discussed openly. Doctors who detected cancer in their patients, often did not tell them, fearing it would send them into a tailspin of despair. They were more likely to disclose the nature of the illness to someone in the family, husband, wife or son, leaving it to that relative to decide whether the patient or others in the family should know. Often cancer stayed secret.

We've taken cancer out of the closets of our minds since then, and with good reason. There are millions of people in North America today going about their lives in their usual ways who have had cancer. More than two million of them have been free of symptoms for five years or more and might be considered cured. For others it is a chronic disease but not a disabling one. Of the 90,000 people in Canada and almost one million in the United States whose cancers will be first diagnosed this year, more than half will be alive five years from now.

To cite percentages or statistics is not to pretend that cancer is no longer a life-threatening disease, nor is it to say that the diagnosis of cancer no longer packs an emotional wallop. Of course it comes as a shock that stuns the mind. One man described it as feeling as if he'd been taken hostage by a madman with a gun and had no idea what to do next.

Yet the fact that over half of all people with cancer can continue their lives, many of them for as long as they would have lived if they had never had cancer, proves to us that cancer is no longer the inevitable death sentence it was at the turn of the century.

In the 1900s few people with cancer lived for long. Even in the 1930s, fewer than one in five patients lived five years. Slowly but steadily since then the odds have been improving—one in four survived in the 1940s, one in three in the 1960s, three in eight in the 1970s and now better than one in two.

Looked at in the context of human history, that is remarkable progress in fifty years. Our minds can register and applaud the achievement. Yet it's not much solace when faced with cancer personally. The possibility of malignancy in our own bodies or those of people we love still chills the soul. Heart disease, it is true, takes many more lives every year—10,000 more last year in Canada alone. But somehow we don't dread heart disease as much. We have the feeling we'd know when trouble was developing in our hearts whereas cancer begins in secret, silently, getting a toe-hold without setting off alarm bells.

Other diseases and the explanations of why they occur seem easier by far to understand. Cancer comes in so many forms it is baffling, defying attempts to predict with any degree of certainty who will get cancer or why.

Usually we think of cancer as one single disease, yet you have probably heard cancer specialists describe it as 100 different diseases, some say 200. In a sense both views are correct. It is a single disease in that it begins within a cell in the body. It is 100 different diseases in that there are many kinds of body cells. These cells belong to various organs and tissues and they have a variety of jobs, just as people in a community have differing occupations. For that reason the symptoms of one kind of cancer may be quite different from those of another kind. Even if two people have cancer in the same organ, say the lung, their cancers may be different types. It depends on which sort of cells became malignant.

Each cell of your body contains its own set of instructions, coded in chemicals, in genes. We may think the micro-chip is a marvel of miniature circuitry, but coiled inside each of our cells are thousands of genes which, if straightened out, would stretch about two meters (six feet). Genes are, in effect, the blueprint from which you were made.

When a cell divides to reproduce itself those instructions are copied and passed on to the daughter cell. Normal cells go about this natural process of growth and renewal in an orderly fashion, seemingly knowing enough is enough. Not so a cancer cell. Its instructions have become garbled and wrong. It passes on those misleading instructions and daughter cells in turn pass them on, until eventually there is an ever-increasing parade of cancer cells, marching to their own drummer, out of harmony with the orchestra of the body. Unlike normal cells, which stop reproducing when needed tissue has been replaced, cancer cells are oblivious to neighbouring cells and overrun the territory, piling up into what we call a tumour. A tumour is not always malignant. Sometimes cells that are not cancer cells stack up in growths called benign tumours. A wart, for example, is a benign tumour and many breast lumps, eight in every ten detected, turn out to be benign. Unless a benign tumour develops in a critical spot where it interferes with a vital organ, it is not a threat to life. Benign tumours stay put. The cells of a malignant tumour do not.

The danger of cancer cells is that as they continue to multiply, they encroach on normal tissue and destroy it. At first, the cells of most kinds of malignant tumours may remain at one location and at that stage the cancer is said to be localized. Detected and eliminated at that point, a cancer may be gone for good. If it is not found and treated, however, it will continue to grow, invading nearby organs and tissue, and cells may break away travelling through the bloodstream or the lymph vessels.

The lymph system has little catch basins, called nodes, at various locations through the body, such as under the arm and in the groin. These may trap breakaway cells. When nodes near a tumour contain cancer cells, confining them to that one region of the body, doctors call the cancer regionalized. If the cells spread to distant parts of the body where they start up new cancers, the cancer is said to have metastasized. Spread of cancer is called metastasis.

Some people think they have two kinds of cancer when a second tumour occurs. Usually they do not. The cells of the secondary tumour are cells from the primary site; that is, if the original tumour was in the breast, a secondary tumour may be in lung or bone but it is made up of breast cells, not lung or bone cells. The treatment required will be different than it would be for lung cancer or bone cancer. In some cases one of the secondary tumours is discovered before the original tumour has been diagnosed. Doctors need to know where the original tumour began in order to plan treatment.

Most of the time there is no definitive explanation as to why one person develops cancer in one part of the body, while another patient has a tumour in another site.

Some kinds of cancer are common, some quite rare. You might think that suggests certain parts of the human body are the most vulnerable. But that isn't the whole story, because patterns of cancer differ in various regions of the world. Epidemiologists, scientists who study diseases in different population groups, have been able to draw a cancer map of the world, demonstrating the global differences. Breast cancer, one of the commonest types in North America and highest of all in the Netherlands, is rare in Japan and China. Liver cancer is not extensive in Western Europe but seen frequently in Greece, most of southeast Asia and in Africa, south of the Sahara desert.

Furthermore, in North America in the past 40 years there have been substantial changes in the incidence of some cancers. Incidence is measured by the number of cases per 100,000 people, adjusted for age. Age is taken into account in comparing one population with another because cancer occurs more frequently in older people. One reason for the increase in the number of people in North America with cancer is that people are living longer.

In North America the most common cancers, apart from skin,

are those of the colon-rectum (large intestine), breast and lung. Skin cancers, other than one kind called malignant melanoma, which is cancer of pigment cells usually in the skin, are often not included in cancer statistics because they are readily detected and cured.

If we look at the picture in Canada thirty to forty years ago we see quite a difference. Stomach cancer was at the top of the list while lung cancer was not among the three commonest kinds. In Canada, as in most western countries, there has been a dramatic decline in stomach cancer. Some scientists have suggested the credit should go to refrigeration. It allows year-round shipping and storage of fresh vegetables and fruits, so we eat more fresh foods and less preserved, salted or pickled foods. Researchers are trying to find out whether fresh vegetables and fruits offer protection against cancer, and, if so, what it is they contain that acts as a shield.

In any case, by 1977, among 42 countries compared, Canada ranked well down the scale in incidence of stomach cancer, 33rd for men and 37th for women, just slightly higher than the United States. Japan had the highest rate of all. Diet appears to be the most likely explanation. Among Japanese people who emigrated to British Columbia in Canada or to the United States, the rate of stomach cancer declined among second and third generation Japanese. However their rate of colon cancer increased.

A study of immigrants in Ontario, a province in which 22 per cent of residents were born outside of Canada according to 1971 census figures, also suggests a change in the rate of stomach cancer among several ethnic populations who came from countries with higher rates. Those rates were changing when studied ten to fifteen years later. While still greater than in Canadian-born people, the incidence among these immigrants was lower than in the countries of their birth. It is possible that as newcomers to this continent adopt North American eating habits, they may also acquire our cancer patterns.

Japan's low incidence of breast cancer and of colon cancer may also turn out to be attributable to diet, in particular to the amount of fat eaten. The Canadian Cancer Society believes there is enough evidence that fat plays a role in cancer to cause it to recommend that we reduce fats of all kinds in our diet. Some medical nutritionists say 30 per cent of calories in fat would be a sensible level. A typical Canadian diet contains over 40 per cent.

Canada has a network of cancer registries across the nation that enable us to keep track of cancer trends. From them it is known that there has been little change in the rates of breast cancer and colon cancer in the country over the past 30 years. Even if the majority of Canadians were to adopt lower fat diets today, we couldn't expect rates of those cancers to change quickly because many of us have been consuming a lot of fat for many years. But in future, among Canadians who grow up eating less fat and possibly more fibre, there may be a decrease in the rates of some cancers.

Quite a different story is the trend in lung cancer. In the early part of this century it was a rare disease. But is has shot up alarmingly in more recent years, first in men and now in women and it is still rising. North American men began heavy cigarette smoking following the First World War. Women took it up after the Second World War. The increase in lung cancer, 25 to 30 years later, reflects the smoking pattern of each sex.

Today, from many studies, we have solid evidence that smoking is a major factor in lung cancer. It is estimated that cigarette smoking is responsible for more than 80 per cent of lung cancers in men and more than 40 per cent in women and it is predicted that lung cancer will, before too long, outstrip breast cancer as the most common cancer in women. In some states it has already done so, according to American Cancer Society surveys.

Figures compiled by Dr. A.B. Miller, director of the epidemiology unit for the National Cancer Institute of Canada, show that 12.4 per cent of cancers in Canada are colon-rectum cancers. Close behind are breast and lung cancers. These three kinds add up to approximately one third of all cases of cancer in Canada. The picture is similar in the United States.

Also relatively common are cancers of the prostate in men; of women's reproductive organs (uterus, cervix and ovary), of the bladder, which is four times more common in men; of the stomach, twice as common in men; pancreas; leukemia and lymphomas including Hodgkin's Disease, which are blood cell and lymphatic tissue cancers.

Changes are being seen in the rates of some of these cancers. Cancer of the cervix in women has decreased substantially since the advent of the Pap test. Named for its discoverer, Dr. George Papanicolaou, it has been widely used as a screening method for more than 20 years. A swab of cells and tissue, taken from the cervix in a quick, painless procedure done in a doctor's office, provides the opportunity to detect cells that are turning malignant before cancer has had a chance to grow into adjoining tissue, or as doctors term it, become invasive. You may have heard this early, pre-invasive stage, referred to as "in situ."

Cancer of the uterus, however, is on the rise. It is not often fatal because it is usually confined to the uterus (womb) which can be removed. While it is unfortunate if it occurs in a young woman wanting a family, the majority of women who get uterine cancer are older, past child-bearing age. One of the possible reasons responsible for more cases of cancer of the uterus is that many women have taken female hormones, estrogens, as treatment for symptoms experienced during or after menopause. Doctors have been urged to prescribe them with much greater caution.

Bladder cancer has been decreasing in women but increasing in men. So far there is not a clear explanation. It has been observed that bladder cancer is more common among long-time smokers and scientists fear we will see a rise in bladder cancer in coming years among women, similar to the upward trend in lung cancer, as more women join the ranks of people who have smoked for more than 30 years.

Cancer of the pancreas is also being detected more often but some scientists suggest this may not be a true increase, rather that is it being diagnosed more accurately as a result of advances in diagnostic technology. Today scanning devices act like windows into the body to aid doctors in locating tumours. Pancreatic cancer has been one of the most difficult malignancies to diagnose and in the past, people may have died of pancreatic cancer before doctors could find out where, in the body, the cancer began.

In the United States a slight increase in the numbers of cancer of the testicles in young men has been reported. It is a relatively rare cancer, occurring in two or three of 100,000 men. Some doctors have speculated the increase might be linked to the use of street drugs but there is no hard evidence yet.

Cancers of the mouth and pharynx (which is the cavity behind the mouth and nose) are far less common in women than in men, comprising one per cent of all cancers in women, but five per cent in men in Canada. Again, smoking is believed to be involved, in particular heavy pipe or cigar smoking, as well as chewing tobacco. There may be other factors and clues may come out of a region in southern China where nasopharynx cancer is extraordinarily frequent. A team of Chinese scientists, sent there to try and uncover the reason, pinpointed certain foods and the way some foods are stored between harvests. But it will take time to teach the people new ways of storage and to see if the scientists are right.

Leukemia is thought by many people to be a childhood cancer, yet ten times as many adults as children develop leukemia and more than half of them are over the age of 60.

Leukemias, which involve abnormal numbers of white blood cells, are much less common then so-called solid tumours, lumps or masses of cells. The majority of cancers begin in tissues that form linings or coverings of organs and passageways. It is called epithelial tissue and this kind of tumour is called a carcinoma. Tumours that originate in connective tissue, bone, muscle and cartilage are called sarcomas. Canada's young hero, Terry Fox, whose attempt to run across the country to raise money for cancer research after he'd lost one leg to cancer won world-wide admiration, had sarcoma of the bone called osteosarcoma. His run had to be discontinued when it was found his cancer had spread to his lungs. Terry was 22 when he began his run in 1980, dipping his artificial right leg into the Atlantic Ocean in St. John's harbour in Newfoundland. He died in June 1981, leaving as his legacy not only more than 25 million dollars he raised for research, but the motivation for many Canadians to take part in an annual fund-raising run in his memory.

The son of American Senator Edward Kennedy, Edward Jr. also had osteosarcoma when he was a teen-ager and lost his right leg in 1973. He was one of the first to be treated with a new version of drug treatment involving super high doses of the drug Methotrexate, followed by an antidote drug to rescue normal cells from destruction. By 1975, he was free of all evidence of disease.

Bone cancer is relatively uncommon, being discovered in about 200 Canadians and 2,000 Americans each year.

When it comes down to the crunch, however, knowing whether the kind of cancer an individual has is common or rare doesn't get to the nub of the matter. With the shock of the diagnosis comes bewilderment and a struggle to comprehend. "Why me? Why did I get cancer?" As one 45-year-old businessman expressed it, "If I knew the cause, then maybe what is happening to me might make some sense."

Wrapped up in the need to know why cancer arises are many questions that produce anxiety. Worries about whether children have inherited a high risk of cancer if the parent is a patient, for example. Or the parents of a child with cancer may be tormented by irrational guilt, fearing they are somehow responsible for letting it happen. They may have vague hopes that if the cause were identified there would be some way of undoing the damage.

In our society we have come to expect science to have answers and to be able to explain the world. It is hard for us to accept that in most cases there is no concrete explanation of why cancer arose in a particular person. Some patients feel angry with cancer scientists for being unable to tell them why they got cancer. True, we know massive doses of radiation can cause cancer and scientists have been able to identify a number of chemical carcinogens (cancer-causing agents) but relatively few of us have been exposed to these known hazards. As researchers make giant strides toward gaining understanding of what takes place in a cell to make it malignant, they have become convinced it takes more than one factor, be it damage by a chemical or some other event.

In most instances, a cancer patient can dismiss some worries from the mind. Inheriting cancer is one of them. You may have heard recently about "cancer genes" being discovered. That can be confusing. Genes, we know, are inherited, passed on from parent to child. But a so-called cancer gene (also called oncogene) is not one that passes cancer from one generation to the next in the way, say, brown eyes are inherited by a daughter from her father. We all have the genes that are being dubbed cancer genes. So do animals and other forms of life. They play an essential role in the growth of the body and we wouldn't be alive without them. They will be explained more fully in the chapter on research. For the moment we need only to be reassured that they do *not* carry cancer from one generation to the next.

You may also have read or heard about "cancer families" in which clusters of cancers occur. That might alarm you. Such families are few in number. Doctors studying them have learned that the explanation seems to lie in the chromosomes. We have 23 pairs of chromosomes inherited from our parents. Our genes are strung along them inside our cells.

One family, with members in Canada and the United States, which has co-operated closely with researchers from both countries, has chromosomes highly vulnerable to damage by radiation even at low doses, putting them at greater risk of cancer. Before scientists found this out some of these people had been treated for cancer with radiation therapy with disastrous results.

In other families, doctors find odd arrangements of certain pieces of chromosomes. In one such family, studied by doctors at the U.S. National Cancer Institute, six members developed highly unusual cancers in both kidneys.

An investigation into the genetics of the family found pieces of two chromosomes had become mixed, with each chromosome having a piece of the other attached. Not all of the family members with this chromosome mix-up developed cancer, so doctors know there must be another factor involved. But it does, apparently, make these people more susceptible to developing cancer.

Doctors suspect a family may be considered a cancer family if unusual cancers occur in more than one young person. But, they say, even several cases of cancer in older members within a family is not an indication the family is at high risk. It is simply that older people make up two-thirds of all cancer patients in North America. For the majority of patients, there is little reason to think their family is more likely than other families to develop cancer.

A second needless worry concerns "catching" cancer from someone who has it. It isn't contagious like measles or the common cold. Viruses linked to human cancers appear to be very rare. The first such virus was discovered in 1980 by Dr. Robert Gallo and his colleagues at the U.S. National Cancer Institute. Called the human T-cell leukemia-lymphoma virus, because it affects a type of white cell called a T-cell, it causes only a small number of cancers in North America. This kind of cancer, however, is more common in Japan and the Carribbean. It appears the virus only spreads from one person to another when other, as yet unknown factors, provide the right conditions. It is not highly contagious.

Other viruses are indirectly involved in cancer although they do not cause it single-handedly. Hepatitis B, a liver disease, is caused by one such virus. People with chronic hepatitis B have been found to be at higher risk of developing liver cancer. It may be that a damaged liver is more prone to cancer. In the last few years a vaccine against hepatitis B has been available and medical scientists are hopeful that preventing the liver disease will bring about a correspondincg drop in the number of cases of liver cancer. Indeed the vaccine has been called "the first cancer vaccine."

There are people who continue to think cancer is spread from person to person. It can be distressing for cancer patients to encounter someone who feels that way, or to find certain acquaintances avoiding them. One woman was hurt and upset when her hairdresser asked her not to come to the beauty salon again after the woman revealed she had been treated for bladder cancer. Today, nine years later, the woman is, as always, beautifully coiffed although she goes to a different hair stylist. Her former hairdresser died of a heart attack two years ago.

When a number of people in one area or working in one industry develop some kind of cancer, it is a tip-off to scientists that something in the environment may be the culprit. For example, skin cancer is common in a country like Australia where many fair-skinned people are exposed to a lot of sunlight. Ultraviolet rays from the sun are to blame. In countries equally sunny but whose people are dark-skinned, skin cancer is not nearly as common. Dark skins contain many more pigment molecules, acting like tiny sunshades to protect genetic material inside skin cells.

Probably the best documented industrial carcinogen is asbestos. It has long been known that asbestos miners are at greater risk of lung cancer than workers in other areas. The odds are even worse if they smoke. The risk to smokers is five times higher than to their non-smoking co-workers and twenty times higher than that of men who do not smoke or work with asbestos. Here we can see what scientists are getting at when they say cancer is a two—or more—step process. It may take both damage to cells from asbestos fibres and something else, such as chemicals in cigarette smoke, to trigger cancer.

Even so, not all asbestos miners, even if they smoke, get lung cancer. Nor, in other occupations, do people who work side by side, exposed to the same chemicals and living similar lifestyles, develop the same disease. Every individual is unique. Your body reacts in its own style to many things. A medicine that the majority of people can take with no ill effects, for example, may make you break out in a rash. You may enjoy a particular food that starts up an allergy in some other person in your family.

Our immune systems, which are body defence mechanisms composed of a variety of white cells, play a key part in how we handle diseases, including cancer. It is known that people whose immune systems have been subdued by certain medical drugs, such as those used to prevent rejection of a transplanted organ, are more vulnerable to cancer. The most publicized example recently is a condition called AIDS, acquired immune deficiency syndrome, in which the immune system of previously healthy young people is suppressed. Among these people, a rare kind of cancer called Kaposi's sarcoma has occurred. It was not cancer that originally made AIDS patients sick but rather that the cancer developed because their immune systems were out of commission.

Some scientists say we all have cells turning malignant regularly but we don't all get cancer because our immune systems are able to identify and destroy aberrant cells before they get out of hand.

None of us can guarantee ourselves freedom from cancer; no place on earth is a cancer-free paradise. But neither is there evidence to support the idea that a cancer epidemic is ravaging North America as some people fear. According to the Canadian Cancer Society, were it not for the rising incidence of lung cancer, we would be winning the fight and the death toll would have dropped substantially as treatments grow ever more effective.

In Canada, with regional cancer treatment centres and national health insurance, Medicare, every patient has access to the same quality of care, care that ranks with the best in the world. The United States has a number of comprehensive cancer centres, designated by the National Cancer Institute, and the American College of Surgeons surveys and certifies hospitals with cancer treatment programmes that meet its standards of quality of care. At the end of this book you will find a list of organizations through which you can obtain information about cancer treatment and rehabilitation services in your area.

But some of the responsibility for their fight to regain health remains in the hands of patients and their families. Patients are not necessarily in hospital throughout treatment and in the next chapters we will look at some of the ways you can help yourself.

Three
Nutrition

YOU WANT TO help your body fight your cancer but there seems to be little you can do. It is frustrating. Is that how you feel? You can do a lot more than you think. You can make sure your body gets the nourishment it needs to withstand the buffeting it must take from treatment and to give it the ingredients to repair or replace healthy tissue.

By eating well you may be able to ward off infections that can crop up when illness makes you more vulnerable to them. Maybe food doesn't sound like a powerful weapon with which to fight cancer but it can be much more important than you suspect.

Maintaining your normal weight, however, is perhaps easier said than done. You may not feel like eating. The disease, the treatment and the emotional upheaval can combine to play havoc with your appetite.

Right now you probably need more calories than you normally eat because your body is using so much energy recovering from surgery, radiation or drug therapy. Weight loss means the body is using up its own stores of fat, protein and other nutrients. Carbohydrates, fat and protein are the three food groups that provide energy and it is important that you eat foods from each group. You require a wide variety of foods to ensure your body gets adequate amounts of vitamins, minerals and other elements.

Not all patients have trouble eating. It depends partly on where the cancer is located and partly on how it is being treated.

Understandably, therapy is more likely to cause nausea in people whose digestive tract is the site of cancer. Nausea is one of the biggest obstacles to eating experienced by cancer patients. In one study of 100 patients, the most common reasons for eating difficulties were found to be stomach and intestinal upsets, fatigue, soreness or dryness of the mouth and just generally seeing food as unappealing.

The patients in the study said it helped them to try and keep an open mind about food. They found that a food that sounded unappetizing one day might sound good the next. They also found on the days when they felt like eating it was a good idea to eat as much as they could, snacking between meals as well as consuming food at meal-times, and getting into their bodies as much nourishment as they could. That way some nutrients were stored for the days when food had no appeal and they couldn't choke it down.

Each kind of therapy can impinge on appetite. Surgery puts stress on the whole body and, as you know if you have had any kind of operation, you only want to eat lightly for a few days afterward. Depending on the surgery, the operation may temporarily interrupt the smooth functioning of body systems. Usually, however, if surgery is the only treatment you have, it isn't long before your appetite has perked up again.

Chemotherapy (drug treatment) and radiation may result in longer-lasting difficulties. Chemotherapy can destroy healthy cells that are frequently dividing to replace themselves, such as cells in the mouth and digestive tract and that may make some foods taste different to you.

To some people certain foods taste metallic, too sweet or too salty. Others, following drug treatments, experience feelings of fullness or cramps after eating only a little. Radiation can also destroy normal cells, although only in the target area that is being treated. But it may cause symptoms that put you off your food.

Each patient is different. Some may experience symptoms early in the course of treatment, some late and some not at all. Usually discomfort abates within a few days after treatment.

Anything that keeps you from eating should be discussed with your physician or nurse or the dietitian on your treatment team. Don't try a home remedy until you discuss it with them to make sure the problem does not require medical attention.

Loss of appetite is sometimes called anorexia. For reasons no one yet fully understands, it can be one aspect of cancer, not just a side-effect of treatment. It can happen to people with cancer who are not undergoing treatment. Some people find it only happens off and on. Others rarely feel hungry.

You may find some foods you used to enjoy no longer taste right. Many patients say they lost their taste for red meat and coffee. You don't need to force down foods that you no longer like. But you do need proteins more than ever to rebuild healthy tissue, inadvertently damaged by treatment. If you previously got a good part of your protein from meat and now often don't feel like eating it, you should replace it with other equally nutritious sources of protein. Cheese, nuts and legumes are some kinds of alternate protein-rich foods.

About a third of the patients who took part in a nutrition study said they no longer enjoyed foods that probably weren't good for them anyway. Candy and fried foods were common examples. These patients also said they tried to avoid foods that caused bloating or gas, such as beans, corn, broccoli and cauliflower.

The foods they most often mentioned as the easiest to eat were fresh fruit and vegetables, dishes made with pasta, milk products, eggs, fish and poultry. All of these foods have good nutritional value and should be part of a well-balanced diet. Some of the patients said they felt a new appreciation for the wisdom of the body. It seemed to be guiding them away from junk foods and toward a healthier diet.

But sometimes weight seems to melt away. One man, undergoing radiation treatment, said he lost 27 pounds in three weeks before he found the solution. He began eating porridge or cream of wheat four or five times a day, consuming a small portion each time. It increased his calories and halted his weight loss.

You may have to experiment with foods to find what tastes good. A number of patients find, to their surprise, they enjoy unsweetened cranberry juice, a drink they seldom if ever, drank before. Others found unsweetened grapefruit or pineapple juice held a new appeal for them.

Patients say it often works better to eat a little but eat frequently during each day. "If you have a lot of nausea it can be awful to think about sitting down to three meals a day," one woman said. "I couldn't face it." She got around the problem by keeping a variety of snacks ready to be nibbled at any time.

Some recent studies have shown that patients who were nauseated by treatment a few times can become "conditioned" to feel sick. The nausea would return when they anticipated the next treatment but before they actually had it. For some, even driving past the treatment centre could bring on nausea. This is similar to the conditioning of Pavlov's dogs. A Russian scientist, Ivan Pavlov, years ago conditioned dogs to produce saliva when a bell rang. They had learned to associate the bell with food because it rang each time they were fed. After a while the dogs drooled to the sound of the bell even when no food was offered. In the same way, the patients' bodies were responding with nausea as a conditioned reaction to treatment.

Some patients suggest that might explain why the sight of certain pieces of crockery or a particular tablecloth seems to trigger their nausea. They had used those items on a dinner table on a day when treatment had made them feel quite sick. You might get clues as to whether you are affected by this kind of body response by observing if you enjoy food more when you change table-settings or eat in a different room of your home.

A number of patients find the smell of cooking ruins their appetites. It's easy enough to stay out of the kitchen if someone else is getting the meals. If you are usually the family cook, somebody else may be willing to take over the job for a while, at least on the days you receive chemotherapy. It is one practical way family members can help.

If you live alone or it is simply not possible for another person to do the cooking, use the days you feel well to prepare meals you can freeze or use canned sauces and soups to make dinners that can be quickly prepared and don't keep you long at the stove.

Try different ways of improving your appetite. Quite a few patients find foods taste better if they are cold or at room temperature instead of hot. If your doctor says an alcoholic drink won't interfere with treatment, a glass of beer or wine may stimulate your interest in food. Going for a walk may make you feel hungrier and keep you away from cooking smells if they are bothersome.

Patients who found they felt full after eating only a small amount say they learned it helped to chew food slowly, to avoid, or at least to cut down on, greasy foods and rich sauces. They also discovered it was better to drink fluids at other times of the day instead of with meals. You will probably be advised to drink more fluid than usual while you are having treatment. It helps your body flush out toxins. Drink fruit and vegetable juices because they supply nutrients as well as just fluid.

Dry foods, such as crackers or toast, may help calm feelings of nausea. Your doctor or nurse may recommend anti-nausea medicines such as motion sickness pills if you are having severe problems with nausea. But be sure to consult them before you take any medication you have on hand at home. Some medicines interact with cancer drugs in adverse ways.

Because the mouth and throat linings are sensitive tissue, patients receiving chemotherapy or radiation may find soreness or dryness interferes with chewing and swallowing. Patients with dentures sometimes find tissue under the teeth becomes irritated. Your doctor or nurse will be able to recommend treatment for mouth problems.

But there are some things you can do to make food go down more easily. A blender may be your best ally to make foods smoother and softer. Mashed potatoes, puddings, milkshakes, creamy cereals and soups slide down fairly readily. Warm, rather than hot foods, are kinder to a sore mouth or throat.

Many people find citrus juices and tomatoes sting and that fruits low in acid, such as bananas, or nectars made from peaches, pears or apricots are preferable. Some find that cold foods like ice-cream, yogurt or popsicles made from fruit juice are soothing.

You may find dryness is eased by rinsing your mouth often. If your house is dry, a humidifier or steam kettle may make you more comfortable. Artificial saliva products are available and you might ask your doctor about prescribing one for you.

Fatigue, also an enemy of appetite, is common in patients. Your body is using so much energy to fight the disease and to recover from treatment, you may feel incredibly weary. People don't feel like eating when they are too tired. Sometimes resting before eating makes a meal more enticing. When you're tired you may not feel like bothering to get dinner ready. In many families, everybody wants to do whatever they can to help and this is a good time to ask. Even a pre-teenager can prepare a simple meal while you rest if you suggest a dish you would enjoy. People of all ages feel good about doing something useful if you let them.

You may learn to predict the times when you'll feel exhausted, possibly the day of certain heavier treatment doses of drugs or on the third or fourth consecutive day of radiation therapy. If friends or neighbours have offered their help, this is a time you can give them the opportunity. Ask to have a supper dish prepared for you. Don't be reluctant to suggest the kind of food you would prefer, nor to explain that you'll be too tired that day for conversation when they deliver the dish. People are sincere about offering to help but often don't know how.

Treatment for some kinds of cancer, involving parts of the digestive system, may interfere with normal digestion and elimination. Nutrition experts say if diarrhoea is a problem, reduce the amount of roughage you eat, use cooked fruits and vegetables instead of raw ones and avoid milk or dishes made with milk until the diarrhoea has stopped. You need fluids to replace what is being lost. With the lost fluids there is also loss of potassium and if you can't get down foods that are high in potassium, fish, meat, potatoes and bananas, it would be wise to discuss potassium supplements with your doctor.

Constipation can result from some drugs, including pain killers. If that is a problem you may need more fibre, fresh vegetables and fruits, whole grain breads and cereals. You might add one or two tablespoons of bran to cereal or casseroles. Hot lemon drinks or prune juice help some patients. You need plenty of liquids. Check with your doctor or nurse before taking laxatives.

Good nutrition helps keep your spirits from sagging as well as helping your body recover. It is well worthwhile perking up your enjoyment of food in any way you can. Flowers on the table, music at dinner time, garnishing your plate with colourful vegetable tid-bits are nice ways to nudge your appetite.

When nothing works, food supplements that provide concentrated sources of protein or calories may be needed to give you adequate nourishment. Commercially-manufactured supplements can substantially increase the nutrient content of a small amount of food. You mix them in. Supplements come in powder or liquid form and can be used in a wide variety of foods. Using these will ensure you are getting balanced proportions of all the essential nutrients. Some brand names are Magnacal, Sustacal and Ensure. Your doctor or druggist can advise you on them. Skim milk powder is also a good source of protein and can be added to whole milk to make puddings or milkshakes.

Usually no particular foods are banned. However, if treatment has lowered your white blood count, making you susceptible to infection, you may be warned to avoid raw eggs. It is always possible that the shell harbours an infective organism. Cooked eggs are fine. You can make an eggnog with a cooked egg, but patients caution that if you are making your own eggnog don't sniff it right away. They have learned the hard way that it smells a bit like sulphur. Wash the shell under running water before breaking the egg into a small pan of boiling water. Cook until the white is firm then put it immediately into a blender with milk, sugar and vanilla.

Begin to think of nutrition as the part of your treatment that you, personally, are responsible for. Keep track of daily calories and kinds of foods eaten to make sure you are not omitting any of the four basic food groups. They are milk and milk products, fruits and vegetables, breads and cereals, and meats and alternate proteins.

Booklets on nutrition have been prepared especially for cancer patients in both Canada and the United States. They contain useful advice and recipes, and are available at some treatment centres or through cancer societies. One booklet, developed at the Health Sciences Centre, Winnipeg, Manitoba, is printed by the Canadian Cancer Society. In the United States a book has been prepared by the U.S. Department of Health and Human Services and may be obtained through the National Cancer Institute, Bethesda, Maryland. The addresses are listed at the back of this book.

In the past, doctors treating cancer patients did not pay great attention to nutrition. Medical schools, typically, gave them scanty training in the subject. But they have become aware how much better well-nourished patients respond to treatment. They have learned that after a few days in bed, even healthy people eating a normal amount of protein, can suffer a protein deficiency. In a study of healthy volunteers, it was found that additional protein was needed by bedridden people to maintain the body's nitrogen balance.

A study of 100 patients undergoing radiation therapy showed half were able to maintain their normal weight. Of those, 44 responded well to treatment, while among the 50 with poor nutrition, only 10 responded as well.

A small percentage of patients who either can't eat or in whom food is poorly absorbed may require nourishment through a vein. Feeding concentrated liquid nutrients via a vein is called intravenous hyperalimentation (IVH). However, eating normally is a superior method of fueling the body and it is important to eat if you possibly can.

Says one doctor, "The importance of maintaining the cancer patient's nutritional status is now recognized as a major part of medical care." Adds another, "Available data increasingly shows that good nutritional status enhances the patient's chance of survival."

That gives you an idea of how much you can do for yourself through nutrition. It's up to you.

Four
Sexuality

IT WOULD BE great if a law could be passed declaring cancer has no business in the bedrooms of the nation. Unfortunately you can't park cancer outside the bedroom door. Physically and emotionally, it can get in your way. Yet almost always sexual pleasure and activity can continue if you want them.

You may have told yourself you'll think about sex later. Right now you're too preoccupied with worrying about sheer survival. Yet before treatment begins, some patients must make decisions that will be of utmost importance to later fertility. Many patients found, as treatment was discussed, they began to speculate on what life would be like if the therapy was successful. Doctors know it is helpful to their patients to provide, at this time, information as to how their sexuality may be affected. If discussion is postponed you may spend many hours needlessly fretting about whether you will ever again feel sexual delight and fearing your partner will look elsewhere.

Sexuality is an inherent part of your personality and your identity. Diagnosis of any serious illness in a previously healthy person is a threat to the self-image that person holds. Maybe you harbour fears your illness will diminish you as a person. If you are nagged by doubts about sexual attractiveness as well, they can play havoc with the mind.

A patient who is still overwhelmed over the diagnosis and by thoughts of the proposed treatment may find it odd for a doctor to bring sex into a discussion. But there are good reasons. When a patient and partner have accurate expectations, much misunderstanding between them can be avoided.

Either the patient or the mate can feel rejected and unloved if the sexual behaviour of the other seems to be changing. Any illness may decrease sexual desire. Often psychological factors are more intrusive than physical ones in an intimate relationship. It has been said that the most important sex organ lies between the ears. The brain plays a bigger role in sexuality than any other part of the body.

For young people who hope to have children some day, it is important that before treatment begins the question of fertility in the future be discussed. Whether or not the patient will be capable of becoming a parent later depends in large part on the type of cancer and the treatment required. It is often impossible to predict with certainty if an individual will become sterile after treatment. But if sterility is a possibility, decisions may have to be made beforehand.

For example, men with Hodgkin's Disease or testicular cancer, both of which more commonly occur in young people, may want to consider sperm banking. This is a process of freezing sperm to preserve it for later use. It can be stored for several years. Should the man and his wife want a child, the sperm would be available for artificial insemination. Although there is no guarantee artificial insemination will bring about a pregnancy, any more than there is by ordinary sexual intercourse, it provides a chance for the couple to have a child who belongs biologically to both parents.

Children have been born to couples who followed this route and the parents are thankful they were informed about sperm banking before the husband underwent treatment for cancer.

Sperm banking is not possible for every patient. Doctors are cautious about raising a couple's expectations. In many cases the disease has already affected the number of sperm or their mobility. Unless sperm can swim vigorously to meet the egg there is slim hope of pregnancy. It can be terribly disappointing for a man to discover his sperm isn't suitable for freezing. Yet if a man is willing to risk that disappointment and has a strong desire to father his own child some day, sperm banking may be worth investigating. Some studies have shown that about four men in ten with Hodgkin's Disease have become infertile as a result of their disease before treatment.

Radiation is the usual treatment for early Hodgkin's Disease. Some men remain fertile despite radiation while others may be temporarily sterile. Doctors say birth control should be practised by a man and his partner during treatment and for about eighteen months after treatment has ended. Radiation may make sperm abnormal and increase the risk of conceiving a child with serious defects. Sperm is produced by the testes which are contained in a sac called the scrotum. The scrotum is protected by a lead shield during radiation treatment to help retain fertility.

It has been learned that it can take up to five years after treatment is complete for a man's sperm count to return to normal. When chemotherapy, as well as radiation, is required to treat Hodgkin's Disease, restoration of fertility and the length of time it takes will depend on the type and dosage of the drugs.

A woman of child-bearing age with any cancer that requires radiation to the pelvic area might want to consider having her ovaries moved out of the target area until treatment is completed. An operation can be performed to attach the ovaries behind the uterus to protect them. The uterus, which is intended by nature to be a shield for an unborn baby, has been found to be an effective barrier to radiation damage. Ovaries contain the eggs a woman will release each month during her fertile years. Until an egg is released, it is contained in a little sac called an ovarian follicle.

Women undergoing treatment for cancer may be advised to take birth control pills. The reason is not only to prevent pregnancy but to help protect the ovaries from the damage of treatment. The pill gives the body the impression the woman is already pregnant and so an egg is not released by the follicle. Follicle cells stay in a resting stage instead of becoming busy preparing to send out the egg. In a resting stage, cells are less apt to be damaged by chemotherapy or radiation.

However, it depends on the kind of cancer a woman has

whether or not she should take birth control pills. The pills contain hormones and some kinds of tumour cells grow better when they are supplied with these hormones. It is crucial that a woman seek advice from her doctor on the method of birth control best for her at this time.

Some women are already pregnant when cancer is diagnosed. That situation demands the special expertise of obstetric counsellors to guide the woman and help her determine whether the pregnancy can continue.

When a man has testicular cancer, he may remain fertile if only one testis has to be removed. If both testes must be removed he will, of course, be infertile. The testes produce the sperm. Treatment may also involve radiation, chemotherapy or surgery to remove lymph nodes in the region. Nevertheless, the probability is high that normal sexual desire, erection and orgasm will not change. For patients who experience a lessening of desire, doctors may suggest levels of the hormone, testosterone, be checked and, if needed, replacement hormones be given. The testes produce hormones as well as sperm.

Men who have lymph nodes removed should be told they may ejaculate little or no sperm. Sometimes that is temporary, but it may take many months for semen to return. As long as the man does not believe semen is synonymous with manhood or that it is important to a woman's sexual pleasure, the lack of semen need not affect his enjoyment of sex. If he holds such beliefs, his partner or physician may be able to debunk the notion and convince him otherwise.

Cancer of the prostate may be accompanied by some changes in sexual performance. The prostate gland produces the fluid ejaculated during sexual intercourse. Radiation treatment can cause some reduction in the amount of semen. But that need not affect orgasm. Sometimes, as a result of radiation, ejaculation may, temporarily, be painful, causing a man to cut down on sexual activity for a while. Otherwise, doctors say, there is no reason to forego sex during the weeks of therapy.

Many people still have the mistaken idea that radiation therapy makes the patient radio-active. Patients have asked if it is all right to kiss their wives or make love, and a few even wonder if they will glow in the dark. There is absolutely no risk to their sex partners and no, they won't glow.

Diagnostic or treatment procedures can, sometimes, cause traces of blood in the ejaculate. It is not unusual or harmful, but may frighten a man if he hasn't been forewarned.

Men who have the prostate removed surgically may need up to six months to overcome erection problems. A high percentage of such patients no longer ejaculate through the penis. Although the sensation a man feels will not be different from normal ejaculation, the semen is released backwards into the bladder. This can be alarming to a man whose physician has not explained it in advance. Doctors call it retrograde ejaculation. It causes no harm to the man and, as mentioned earlier, the absence of semen does not diminish the pleasure of his partner.

At one time, doctors did not give much consideration to impotency in prostate cancer patients. In those days it was assumed that interest in sex vanished in older people. The majority of prostate cancer patients are over the age of sixty. But now it is recognized that age is not an indication of whether a man is sexually active. Because cancer of the prostate is the second most common cancer in men, after lung cancer, and because treatment today offers a high probability of success, more attention is being paid to preserving sexual ability.

Doctors often encourage a patient to try love-making after he's recovered from prostate surgery, but not to be discouraged or impatient. Wait and see if erection and orgasm return without striving too hard for sexual intercourse, the doctors advise. There is much joy in holding and touching without intercourse necessarily being a couple's goal. "I've been impotent since my treatment and we haven't been able to have intercourse," said one man who had prostate cancer. "But holding my wife close at night, cuddling and talking to each other means a lot. My wife says it doesn't matter a whit to her that we don't have intercourse. She makes me know I'm still a man."

Sexuality is much more than sexual intercourse. Wrapped up in it is how we see ourselves and whether or not we believe others see us as a person worthy of love. To feel good about yourself as a man or a woman enriches your life and you can do that without noteworthy sexual performance. Sexuality is just as important to a person who is celibate as to anybody else.

One factor in self-esteem is the image a person has of his or her body. For some people, physical appearance is terribly important. For them, loss of a body part or hair loss as a result of treatment is devastating. "You don't have any idea how much hair is a part of your identity until you lose it," one patient said. "Seeing clumps of hair coming out is like seeing yourself falling apart before your very eyes." At the time it isn't much consolation to know that hair loss is generally temporary and regrowth may begin even before treatment is completed.

If you have been told you might experience hair loss after treatment begins, you may find it less upsetting if you are prepared by having a wig or toupee ready. Some people prefer hats. One teen-ager simply wore his ski toque, indoors and out. For intimate moments or hospital stays, many women find a snug-fitting turban with natural looking hair bangs attached, is most comfortable. "You can imagine what it does to love-making if you're wearing a wig and are worried about it staying on straight," one woman confided. "You know if it gets askew you're going to look ridiculous."

The way a body change affects a person's sexuality can depend a great deal on the partner's reaction. It is especially true for women who have mastectomies. A woman who has a breast removed may feel less desirable and torment herself, agonizing over what her lover is thinking. Even women with long and stable marriages say they suffered doubts about themselves and needed repeated reassurances from their husbands.

Mastectomy Visiting Service is a programme through which women who have learned to adjust to mastectomy help other such women. Some of the visiting volunteers say the partner of a mastectomy patient is often unsure about when to resume sex. He may assume the woman is not ready yet and so doesn't mention the subject. At the same time, the woman may begin to think he no longer finds her sexually attractive. "When there is no communication, valuable time in the recovery process is lost," says a guide book produced by the organization called Reach for Recovery. "The sooner you can share your feelings, the sooner you will resume normal relationships."

In one Canadian study on the quality of life after mastectomy in which 166 women participated, 13 per cent said they had no further sexual interaction with their husbands or lovers following surgery. Half no longer allowed their partners to see them naked. Several of the women's marriages had ended. The study found that most of the problems were fostered by lack of communication between partners. Some simply never mentioned the surgery to each other at all. If only they had been able to talk it out, they might have discovered the woman's surgery made no difference to their feelings for each other.

Single women who have mastectomies sometimes resign themselves to life without a love relationship. It is a door they need not close. Many women have later met and married men whose love didn't waver when they learned of the breast surgery.

Some studies have found that women patients often fare better emotionally in dealing with cancer because they are better able to express openly their fears and desires than are men. A man who considers it a weakness to talk about his anxieties or who equates his manliness with physical strength or with being the family breadwinner, may have a bitter struggle adjusting emotionally. Even with no physical reason for disruption of his sex life, his illness may make him feel emasculated and unable to fulfil his sexual needs. It may not even be clear in his own mind what is happening to his emotions. If he has customarily been the one to initiate sex, the woman who loves him may not know what to do. Will he feel worse if she suggests they make love and he can't respond? She doesn't want to contribute to his flagging sense of masculinity.

When there have been problems in a marital relationship before cancer was diagnosed, they may become magnified under the new stress of illness. Yet, some patients say it was only after cancer forced them to talk to each other more openly and they gained insights into each other's feelings that they were able to unload old grudges and move toward real closeness.

Even in the best of relationships, however, treatment and

illness may interfere with sexual activity. One of the biggest obstacles is fatigue. It is normal for fatigue to cause a decrease in sexual desire but it won't last for ever. Much of a patient's fatigue is due to the treatment.

For the time being, a couple may need to plan when they will make love. This will take a little getting used to for couples who have always acted spontaneously. Patients may find a rest before having sex will recharge their batteries. Some say they schedule sexual activity for a day in the week they know they'll be least exhausted. For example, some people receiving radiation five days a week say they feel relatively well on Monday and Tuesday, but fatigue sets in on Wednesday. Usually week-ends are treatment free, giving normal tissue a chance to recover. Energy may be high by Sunday evening. Your fatigue pattern may be different and it will take a little time to find out what works best for you.

People receiving chemotherapy, after a short time on the treatment regime, learn when they can expect to be least tired. A few people think, wrongly, that chemotherapy can be transmitted from patient to partner and that sex should be avoided during treatment. One woman was afraid she would lose her hair from the strong drugs her husband was taking if they made love. It is simply not so.

Certain side-effects of chemotherapy may force sex to be put on hold temporarily because of discomfort to the patient, but not because of any hazard to the partner. Some patients develop small sores in the mouth or vagina. They are not contagious. They are caused by the impact of the drugs on sensitive tissue. These sores may make sexual activity painful.

Pain of any kind has an effect on a person's sexual response. A partner may be so afraid of causing pain to a patient, his or her own desires are set aside and sex is avoided. Yet the patient, not knowing why, may feel their love is fading and be forlorn. If allowed to, cancer, with its many ramifications, can drive wedges between people who love each other.

When a patient has continuing pain, a couple should figure out together the best time for love-making. It may be when pain relief medication is at its most effective or when pain has abated after a session of relaxation therapy. Pain control will be discussed more fully in the next chapter. The pair may also find ways, such as placement of pillows, to make the patient more comfortable. Some people, particularly if they experience shortness of breath, have found a water bed is the answer because less exertion is required during sexual intercourse. Others try different positions which prevent weight being put on the patient.

Patients whose treatment reduces blood count and hence increases susceptibility to infection will need advice from their doctors about sexual activity. If the risk is high, the doctor may suggest sex be postponed for a while. In particular, if such patients include anal intercourse in their sexual repertoire, the doctor may caution against it for the time being.

It is natural for people to have questions about the impact of cancer treatment on sex. Not every doctor is skilled at discussing it. If you feel your doctor is not providing the information you need or if you don't feel comfortable discussing sexual problems with your regular doctor, you might ask to be referred to an expert. At some treatment centres, nurses or psychologists are more experienced in sex counselling than doctors treating cancer. Your sexuality to too important to your well-being to be ignored. The day is gone when patients could expect to be told, "Don't worry about sex, you're lucky to be alive."

"Cancer has a broad impact on sexuality and it can pull people apart when they really need closeness," says one nurse who has been involved in much research into human values. "When people are sick, they need demonstrations of affection. They need hugging and touching even more than they need sexual intercourse. We know touch and love have healing powers."

The nurse says some patients increase sexual activity, reporting it reduces stress and makes them feel better. There may be a physical explanation, she adds, because brain chemicals called endorphins, which are the body's own tranquillizers and pain relievers, are released.

Five
Controlling pain

EMBEDDED IN THE public's view of cancer is the belief that pain is cancer's constant companion. It isn't so. Pain is rarely a symptom of early cancer and some patients never experience it at all. In one long-term study in Melbourne, Australia, involving a large number of cancer patients treated at two hospitals, it was found that 25 per cent had no physical pain and another 50 per cent experienced only pain that could be easily relieved.

We think of pain as being a bad thing. Overall, it is extremely useful protection. It is how nature tells us to get our hand off that hot stove. Quickly! Without it we could unwittingly damage our bodies mercilessly.

But it would be nice if we were equipped with a button that could shut off pain once we've received the message. Since we haven't a button, the next best thing is to drown out the message or stop it from getting through to the brain. There are many ways to go about this.

When pain does occur, it can be as demanding of attention as a cranky two-year-old child. It refuses to be ignored and you can't concentrate on anything else until it is relieved.

There are a variety of reasons cancer may cause pain. The tumour may be pressing on a nerve. It may be blocking a blood vessel so tissues are in short supply of blood and are sending distress signals. Sometimes treatment, rather than the disease, can cause pain. Following surgery, for instance, as after any operation, the incision usually causes soreness.

Tissues, damaged by radiation or chemotherapy during the process of destroying cancer cells, sometimes hurt because they are swollen or inflamed.

Pain is a very subjective sensation. We have different pain thresholds, i.e. differing levels of how much pain we can tolerate. In some people, pain signals seem to get through louder and clearer than in others. Only you can know what you feel and it isn't always easy to describe the degree of pain to somebody else. If you can give your doctor a precise picture of your pain it helps to determine how to treat it.

The doctor will need to know how often you feel pain and how long it lasts. That's fairly straightforward. You may be able to point to the spot that hurts, although sometimes pain is diffuse and seems to be here, there and everywhere. From other experiences with pain you have had in the past, you may know what works for you. Discuss it with your doctor. Don't use home remedies without asking your doctor about them first. Try to take note of anything that seems to make your pain worse and see if it can be avoided. Sometimes the anticipation of pain is almost worse than the actual sensation. An injection, for example, causes certain people more discomfort from the expectation of pain than from the shot itself.

Your doctor will want to know if your pain is worse now than it was earlier. It's not always easy to remember the severity of yesterday's pain. At some pain clinics people are advised to make up a pain scale—possibly one to five, ranging from no pain to severe pain—to help them rate the degree of pain. It is a useful way of determining how effective pain relief measures are when you use the scale to rate the degree of pain before and after treatment.

Pain and distressing emotions can set up a vicious circle. Pain seems worse when you are suffering anxiety or depression. Conversely, such feelings are made deeper by pain. Some patients found that when they were able to talk out their feelings and fears with a family member, clergyman, physician or another patient, it rid them of pent-up worries and also lessened physical pain.

When you are tired pain can seem worse and be harder to bear.

Your body is using up so much energy fighting the disease and restoring itself after treatment, you are bound to suffer fatigue. Patients have said they felt better when they were made aware it was tiredness that made their pain seem more severe. They had been fearful it was an indication they were becoming sicker.

Pain isn't always an indication that matters are worsening. Consider, for instance, the pain people can feel from a part of the body that is no longer there. A woman who has had breast surgery may feel pain coming from the breast that has been removed. This hard-to-understand type of pain is called phantom limb pain. Some scientists say small regions in our brains are devoted to each part of the body, as if a map of the body is drawn on the brain. It can take time for this map to be altered when the body has been changed. The regions of the brain devoted to a breast or a leg that has been removed may be sending signals of alarm because they are not getting the customary information from that part. Something is wrong. The pain is quite real and calls for relief measures as much as any other pain.

Some people try to bear pain for as long as possible before taking pain-relief medication. That usually isn't wise. It is easier to control pain by preventing it than by overcoming it once it has built up and become unendurable. Your doctor will plan a regular schedule of medication to keep pain at bay. In the past, it was more common for doctors to order pain drugs "as needed." Now they know it is more effective not to wait until relief is required but to keep pain under control all the time. Usually lower doses are needed to keep on top of the pain than if you wait until pain is intense. Not having to endure pain until the drug starts to take effect, is a further advantage.

Pain relievers, also called analgesics, may be prescription drugs or they may be over-the-counter medicines that do not require a prescription. The most common pain killer you can buy without a doctor's prescription is ASA (acetylsalicylic acid), often called aspirin. (In Canada Aspirin is a brand name restricted to one manufacturer's product but in the United States the word aspirin can mean any ASA product.) Almost as common is acetaminophen.

Some patients who, over the years, often take ASA don't realize how important it is to ask their doctors before using it when they are being treated for cancer. For certain patients, ASA can be harmful. ASA acts on blood-clotting mechanisms, lengthening the time it takes blood to clot. Certain kinds of chemotherapy can cause bleeding and patients receiving such drugs should avoid ASA. Ask your physician before taking ASA products. Never take ASA prior to surgery. It could cause surgical wounds to bleed excessively.

If your doctor has given approval for you to use ASA, you can expect it to reach its peak effect in about 45 minutes and to last three or four hours. ASA acts at the site of pain rather than in the central nervous system and it doesn't affect mood. It reduces swelling from inflammation and can be particularly helpful for those whose pain stems from swollen tissue. But it can cause stomach upsets. Many pain relief products contain ASA and if your doctors says you should definitely not use ASA, be wary of combination products. Consult your pharmacist to make sure you are not unknowingly buying products containing ASA.

Some people may develop a ringing in their ears after taking ASA for several days. It is usually an indication the dose should be cut down or the drug stopped. In some cases it is a forewarning of more serious adverse effects. Any other symptoms such as sweating, dizziness, nausea or rapid breathing should be reported right away to your doctor.

Acetaminophen is equal in its pain-easing effectiveness to ASA, but it does not reduce swelling. Because it doesn't increase bleeding, some patients who should not use ASA can safely use acetaminophen. But prolonged use, especially if acetaminophen is taken daily in large doses, may have an adverse effect on liver or kidneys. You should discuss its use with your doctor before taking it.

In general, doctors consider it prudent for patients to take single-drug products rather than combination-type pills. There is no evidence that plain ASA or acetaminophen is less effective than products to which other substances are added. The extra ingredients are sometimes the cause of unwanted effects.

You may think simple headache tablets are pretty feeble pain fighters for a person who has cancer. It can be a surprise to find ASA or acetaminophen is all you need. They are stronger than most people realize. Studies have found that for many people they work as well as prescription drugs such as codeine or meperidine (Demerol).

If you have been given a prescription pain drug, ask your doctor whether you should continue to take non-prescription drugs as well. The doctor may want you to do so because it means you will require smaller doses of the prescription drug or because the two kinds of drugs are directed at pain from different directions and double the pain relief. On the other hand, some prescription drugs already contain ASA or acetaminophen and if you continue to take additional doses of them you may be getting higher than safe levels.

Prescription drugs include both narcotics and non-narcotics. Codeine, morphine and heroin are narcotics but so are a number of other drugs, such as Demerol, Dilaudid, Percodan and Numorphan that you might not be aware are in the same category. While heroin is available to patients in Britain, in North America it was banned in 1955, in accord with an agreement with the World Health Organization and the United Nations Commission on Narcotics. Since then heroin has been the subject of much controversy and medical opinion is split over whether it should be available to combat cancer pain.

On the one hand, it is argued that heroin is broken down into morphine in the body and that morphine or heroin are equally effective when given properly. On the other hand, heroin is more soluble and can be given in smaller amounts of fluid. For people who require very large doses or those for whom repeated injections are extremely painful, heroin may bring relief that morphine cannot provide.

The real fear of reinstating heroin as a legal, medical drug is that some of it would be diverted into illegal channels and become a supply for heroin addicts. But those who consider heroin an indispensable weapon against pain for some cancer patients or people who are terminally ill, believe suffering people should not be deprived of it because of public worries about addicts. How extensively heroin will come to be used against cancer pain in the future remains to be seen.

At one time there was widespread fear that giving narcotics to relieve pain posed a risk because the patient might become addicted. Well-meaning nurses and doctors withheld narcotics from patients in pain if they suspected the patients were becoming dependent on the drugs. Gradually, opinion changed. First because it was senseless to fear addiction in a person who was dying and second, because a number of studies showed that people in severe pain who were given narcotics did not often become addicted. When their pain was gone, so was their need for the narcotics. Only in rare cases were patients unable to give them up quite readily.

Family or friends, however, may be unaware of these findings. Some patients said their relatives became alarmed when the patients took narcotics for any length of time. If this becomes a troublesome issue in your family, the physician under whose supervision you are taking the drugs should be willing to explain the situation to your family.

Marijuana, which many people think of as a recreational drug, has also found a place in cancer therapy. The U.S. National Cancer Institute has recommended that an ingredient of marijuana, delta-9-tetrahydrocannabinol (THC), be made available to patients who suffer severe nausea and vomiting as a result of chemotherapy, if standard anti-nausea drugs will not help. A drug of this kind, a chemical cousin of THC, called nabilone, is available in Canada. It is not a narcotic.

Sometimes nausea is the result of pain and will go away when pain is relieved. In other cases, narcotics used to ease pain may cause nausea for a few days.

You may hear of Brompton's Cocktail. It is the name used for a mixture of ingredients, including a narcotic, given to patients to drink to relieve pain. Brompton's Cocktail was first used in England and contained heroin or morphine. Now ingredients vary from place to place, but typically the mixture includes one substance to counteract sleepiness, another to counter nausea, flavouring and a narcotic.

Certain narcotic-like drugs can work against other narcotics. You must understand explicitly when and how to take your drugs if you have prescriptions for more than one. Talwin is one widely-used drug that should not be taken in conjunction with a narcotic. If it is, a patient may experience nasty flu-like symptoms.

It takes skill and expertise in pharmacology for a physician to keep pain from breaking through into a patient's awareness but in most treatment centres pain control today is far more effective than ever before. Furthermore, new techniques for easing pain have been added to the drugs.

A number of patients have found they can help rid themselves of much pain by methods which do not involve drugs. Relaxation, for example, by reducing tension in the body, may make other anti-pain weapons work better. It usually takes at least a couple of weeks to train yourself to make use of relaxation techniques and some people have found they needed to take lessons in relaxation before they discovered any benefits. If you cannot attend a course, you might inquire about tape-recorded instructions that outline, step by step, relaxation techniques.

Another method some patients find useful is distraction. It may help while you wait for pain medication to take effect. Some people become so skilled at distracting themselves away from their pain they can ease even severe episodes. Anything that absorbs your attention fully can do the trick. Young people say often they can drown out pain by blasting their head with loud music. A gripping book or TV show might be more your style.

Hot or cold packs or massage may also lessen pain. It is probable that temperature signals and pressure messages travel on the same nerve pathways to the brain as pain. When pain tries to get through, the line may be busy. Do not, however, use these measures on areas that have received radiation, because skin and tissue are often extraordinarily sensitive after radiation and could be easily damaged.

Transcutaneous electric nerve stimulation, TENS, a device that electrically stimulates the skin and blocks pain, has been found useful by some people. It gives a tingling sensation that gets in the way of pain signals.

Biofeedback techniques, acupuncture and hypnosis are other methods that have sometimes proven helpful. There are medical

Narcotic drugs commonly used for pain control

Drug (Brand names)	How given Dosage range	Duration of effect	Comment
Butorphanol Tartrate (Stadol®)	Injected 1.5 to 2.5 mg.	3-4 hours	May cause withdrawal symptoms if taken while using other narcotics
Codeine phosphate	By mouth 30 to 60 mg.	3-4 hours	
Hydromorphone (Dilaudid®)	Injected 1.5 to 4 mg. By mouth 2 to 4 mg.	3 hours	May also be given by rectum
Levorphanol (Levo-Dromoran®)	Injected 1 to 4 mg. By mouth 1 to 3 mg.	4-6 hours	
Methadone	Injected 5 to 10 mg. By mouth 5 to 15 mg.	6-8 hours	Caution: build-up effect
Morphine	Injected 2.5 to 15 mg. By mouth 8 to 20 mg.	3-4 hours	Preferred drug
Nalbuphine (Nubain®)	Injected 10 to 20 mg.	3-6 hours	May cause withdrawal symptoms if taken while using other narcotics
Oxymorphone (Numorphan®)	Injected 1 to 1.5 mg.	4-6 hours	May be given by rectum
Oxycodone (Percodan®, Percocet®)	By mouth 5 to 10 mg.	3-4 hours	Contains ASA Acetaminophen
Meperidine (Demerol®)	Injected 50 to 100 mg. By mouth 50 to 150 mg.	2-3 hours	Short duration use discouraged
Pentazocine (Talwin®)	Injected 30 to 60 mg. By mouth 50 to 100 mg.	3-4 hours	Many side-effects. Use discouraged.

doctors who have become knowledgeable about the use of acupuncture to whom your own physician might refer you if he or she doesn't have the expertise. It involves inserting fine needles into the skin at specific points. In China and other oriental countries acupuncture has long been used, even as an anaesthetic during surgery. No drugs are given and patients stay awake yet are comfortable during the operation.

Biofeedback involves learning to control, with the mind, certain body functions. For example, people can learn to raise the temperature of their hands, improving circulation, or lower their own blood pressure or decrease muscle tension, by manipulating their thoughts. A machine measures and feeds back to you information about what is happening in your body so you know when you are achieving control. In most large cities there are practitioners who specialize in biofeedback.

A number of physicians teach self-hypnosis to control pain or hypnotize a patient to implant the suggestion that pain will not be felt. Some patients say it has reduced their anxiety knowing they can use self-hypnosis to combat pain. The strategy of teaching hypnosis typically requires a patient to attend regular sessions to learn and practise the technique. It isn't magic but it may allow a patient to substitute a pleasant feeling for pain or to move the pain to another spot in the body where it is tolerable.

When pain is extreme and no effective measures to control it can be found, doctors may suggest radiation or surgery to cut a nerve. Radiation, in some cases, can rid patients of pain even when it cannot successfully treat their cancer.

Most large communities now have pain clinics located in hospitals or run by doctors with particular expertise in pain control. Your doctor might refer you to such a clinic where a pain control regime, possibly involving a combination of methods, can be devised for you.

A lot of patients say they tortured themselves with dread of the day when their cancer would cause them excruciating pain, only to learn the agony of anxiety had been needless. Their pain could be managed effectively. You can be reasonably confident that should you have pain, ways have been developed to erase it.

Six
Families are human too

FEW OF US live in isolation from our fellow man. Humans require for emotional health others to whom they matter. Whether or not they are related, the circle of people who care about you is your family. When we talk about families in this chapter, these are the people we mean. You don't have to have a spouse or children or parents for this section to apply to you.

When a person develops cancer, the family feels the impact. Often they are under stress as great as the patient's. There may be changes in their lives that they had never anticipated. Cancer can turn a family unit topsy-turvy and restoring its equilibrium will be a task of impressive magnitude. Many people facing cancer with those they love find it becomes possible to cope only when they better understand themselves. Such understanding does not come quickly. First there is the adjustment to the acute shock of the diagnosis which is often as heart-wrenching for the family as for the patient.

Usually practical arrangements have to be made. Temporarily, the place the patient filled in the family may have to be taken over by someone else. A substitute homemaker may be required to look after the children while their mother is in hospital or making daily visits to a treatment centre. A wife may have to take on the role of decisive head of the family, assuming responsibilities her husband has always carried. A grandmother, looked after by her husband before he got cancer, may need to move in with her daughter. Each family has its own situation.

It is natural for families whose lives have been disrupted to long for what used to be. Frequently they idealize the former situation. They begin to imagine family life before cancer as idyllic, forgetting that a typical day was peppered with frustrations, annoyances and conflicts. There is a tendency to go through an "if only" syndrome, when people compulsively go over and over in their minds events that preceded the diagnosis, trying to pinpoint things that might have been altered to prevent what has happened. Family members may start blaming themselves. Counsellors say self-recrimination within a family is almost universal.

One social worker explains that often it is less disturbing to people to find someone to blame, even themselves, than to accept the realization that life is uncertain and reasons for disease inexplicable. It may seem irrational for people to blame themselves. The social worker says one instance that stands out in her mind is the case of a man whose wife had a brain tumour. He had convinced himself his wife's tumour was his fault because she had driven him everywhere some months earlier when his broken leg was in a cast. Obviously, there was no connection. Why did he cling to his belief?

Illogical as blaming oneself might be, it can be less frightening than not feeling in control of one's life. Yet when the husband was persuaded he was in no way responsible for his wife's tumour, he had more energy to use constructively for the task of looking after his wife and himself.

If you are caring for a person with cancer, you will almost inevitably find you are reproaching yourself sometimes. Even if you don't go so far as to blame yourself for the patient's illness, you may resent the disruptions in the home being caused by the disease. You might focus your resentment on the patient once in a while. Knowing this is unfair, you feel guilty and rake yourself over the coals.

You may feel disgusted with yourself for being irritated by the patient's behaviour or because you sometimes feel angry with the patient. We all have negative feelings, at times, toward those we love. It is impossible not to feel some ambivalence toward those we care about most. If you don't understand that such feelings are normal, whether or not a loved one is ill, it can make you feel unduly rotten about yourself.

You may expect of yourself a saintliness of thought that is humanly impossible. Some people are horrified to discover that, for a fleeting moment, they wished the patient would die and end the ordeal. It's not that they love the patient less. It is natural for the human brain to search for every possible avenue of escape from distress. It is a problem-solving mechanism, similar to a computer search for data, scanning the potential solutions. To be aware of an idea crossing your mind is not the same thing as really wanting it to happen.

Psychologists, however, say there is a danger. Under strain, a person can experience the re-emergence of the irrational beliefs of childhood. Small children, typically, think they are the centre of the universe and that whatever they wish for will happen.

Without consciously realizing it, an adult may revert to that infantile belief. Suppose such a person has had flash through his mind a wish for the patient's death and the patient worsens. The guilt can be awesome. By understanding why such a thought could enter your head, you may protect yourself from guilt you cannot bear to live with.

More commonly, family members may begin to question if they really possess the qualities on which they have based their self-esteem. They may have feelings that shake their image of themselves as "good" people. One daughter became highly disparaging of herself because, she said, she was worrying about failing her year at university as a result of missing classes to look after her sick mother. "How can I begrudge her my time when she has cancer?" the daughter asked. "What kind of a daughter would do that?" She felt miserable although from the perspective of others she was a devoted daughter, providing all the tender attention possible.

You cannot shove your own needs and those of others in the family right out of the picture. You will be doing the patient no favour if you try, because eventually you will be unable to be genuinely caring and cheerfully supportive. Nor will it do the patient any good to have you reproaching yourself internally for not doing more than can be reasonably expected.

You will need to assess your own limitations and strengths and get assistance when you require it, either from other family members and friends or by means of outside help. Over the long haul of weeks of treatment you may not be able to hold up if you don't allow yourself to put your own needs first now and then. If the patient is housebound, you might think it isn't right for you to go out and enjoy yourself periodically when the patient cannot. Give yourself permission to take a little time for yourself. Do not listen to accusations of selfishness from yourself or from others. Healthy members of a family have rights that must not be sacrificed to the disease. If cancer is allowed to devour the time others need for rest and relaxation, it may destroy the refuge a family provides for the patient. Everybody, including the patient, must have days that are filled with more things than paying attention to cancer.

In some families, a patient who is capable of participating in normal household activities and sharing responsibilities is turned into an invalid. It's done with love in an attempt to protect the patient. Since there is nothing they can do about the cancer, families do everything for the patient. But the net result may be that the patient ends up feeling more helpless than ever and more focused on the disease. "If I didn't have cancer I'd be washing the dishes," a woman thinks to herself. "I'm not even good for that any more."

A wife, trying to shelter her husband, took over the family finances. "Fat help that was," she says. "It made him feel I thought he was mentally incompetent on top of everything else."

Some patients are quite capable of speaking up for themselves and reject a take-over of their usual tasks or responsibilities when they feel well enough to carry on. Families can best help by heeding their wishes and even encouraging them to preserve their ordinary routines. Yet sometimes a person, especially a man who saw himself as the family strongman, is so badly shattered by the realization of his vulnerability, he lets himself become dependent to a needless degree. Unintentionally, his family may have led him deeper into the emotional mire.

In some instances a marriage partner, frightened for the patient, restricts pleasures the patient might have enjoyed. One husband insisted his wife give up singing with a community choir. "It's too hard on her," he said, although his wife loved it. The husband did not admit it to himself, but his determination to "protect" her stemmed from fear he would never be able to forgive himself if she died and he hadn't kept her safe beside him.

In certain families internal conflicts existed long before cancer was diagnosed. For them the difficulties may be compounded. One woman who had been intending to ask for a divorce couldn't bring herself to leave her husband when he developed cancer. Yet she felt angry and resentful toward him for thwarting her plans. In addition, she began to believe that her desire to end the marriage had somehow brought on his disease. Eventually she became seriously depressed and in need of psychiatric therapy.

In other families adult children, who have had long-standing feelings of alienation from their parents, may suffer a bitter sense of disappointment when a parent develops cancer. It may seem the parent never fully loved and accepted them and now time appears to be running out. It is too late to build the kind of relationship they yearned for deep in their hearts. They may never have the chance to win the parent's approval. Yet sometimes cancer is the catalyst that enables the gap between parent and grown child to be bridged. For the first time, a son or daughter may be able to risk feeling rejection by the parents and be willing to express cravings for the parents' love. It can become a time of emotional mending for both.

Even in families with the best of interpersonal relationships, at times as treatment continues, it is hard to remember the patient is still the same person you love. Bitterness and irritation shown by the patient may get you down when you are doing your best to nourish him or her emotionally. You have to keep reminding yourself that the disease, treatment and uncertainty all conspire to twist moods, creating a mental wringer for the patient. "Learning to live with cancer is clearly no easy task. Learning to live with someone else's cancer may be even more difficult," one family counsellor says.

You should expect the deep fatigue that results from treatment to cause irritability. Therapy may make patients feel sicker than they felt at the time of diagnosis and their discouragement may intensify. Returning again and again to the treatment centre or doctor's office to undergo treatment that brings no immediate improvement and may even knock the patient for a loop physically, may seem futile and depressing.

There will be days when you feel you aren't of any help to the patient at all. Your attempt to show affection may be pushed away. Whatever you say seems wrong. Treatments often affect the emotions as well as the body and cause swings in mood. But even when you know that and understand, you may wonder how long you can keep up your own morale.

Those who have gone through this emotional battering advise families to grab hold of the good days, using the times the patient feels well to do special things together. Share smiles and dreams, they say. Do whatever adds zest to your day. Have dinner at a favourite bistro, invite in old friends for a game of cards, or go to an outdoor concert under the stars. They say you will be surprised how much your spirits will recuperate. Benefits will flow from the fun you have had together, spilling over into the awful days and offsetting them.

Treatment will end, and free of symptoms or with the disease under control, the patient's familiar self will bounce back. You may be amazed at how much you have grown emotionally and in knowledge and understanding of yourself and of the person you love.

Seven
Facing the world

WHEN FRIENDS, NEIGHBOURS or near strangers learn of your cancer, their reactions may astound you. They can warm your heart or dismay you, make you feel tearful or outraged. Many patients and family members say they were quite unprepared for the way other people would respond.

"For the first while I got more attention than I'd ever experienced in my life," one woman said. "I had cards from folks I hadn't heard from in years or scarcely knew. It was rather exciting. Then it was all over. I thought this is what it must be like to be a widow. Everybody rallies around you and then they're gone. You are alone."

Another patient who experienced a similar flurry of concern and then virtual silence found that, as the months went by, when he ran into old acquaintances the look in their eyes seemed to say, "What? Are you still alive!" To the man it seemed as if they were uneasy to meet him. "They'd paid their respects to the dead man and here he was walking around," he said.

A large segment of society is still unaware of the fact that cancer today may be a chronic disease. "I've had cancer for seven years and I sure wish people would treat me like they would if I had heart disease or diabetes," said a feisty 58-year-old woman. "I could be worse off if I'd had a bad stroke but nobody ever seems to think of that."

People with cancer often feel very much alone. You may feel the world has backed away from you. Some friends fade over the horizon, they stop calling or visiting. Patients say they learned they often had to take the initiative and reach out to friends.

"What you project is what you get back," explained one man. "If you attitude is 'Hey, I can handle it,' other people treat you in a way that shows they too think you are okay. That's what I found."

Lots of people do not know if you want to mention your disease. They may carefully avoid asking how you are feeling in case the question would upset you. You might get the impression they don't care how you are. That's seldom true. Far more often they don't know what to say and saying nothing seems safer than blurting out the wrong thing.

"I was really hurt when a couple of my friends didn't call me when I got home from hospital," said one woman. "But when I called them and said I guessed they'd realized how sick I'd been but that I was coming along fine now and felt like seeing my friends, I was touched by the relief in their voices. Once I'd broken the ice they were all right and started phoning me again."

Certain people have such dread of cancer they will avoid you despite your attempts to re-establish contact. In a letter to advice columnist Ann Landers a while ago, a woman wrote of her obsession. She'd had no past experience to account for it. "I know cancer isn't contagious but I am so afraid of it I can't bring myself to visit my neighbour," she wrote. Her neighbour had had a mastectomy.

Although sometimes fear of cancer stems from ignorance, in some people it is a phobia. People with phobias, such as claustrophobia (fear of enclosed places), cannot get over them by telling themselves their fear is groundless. The panic they suffer is beyond their control. If you have friends who are cancerphobics, they will withdraw from you despite themselves. You will undoubtedly feel badly but there is nothing you can do. Try to save yourself hurt by realizing it is not you, as a person, who is being shunned.

Sometimes patients themselves are the ones who withdraw from their social group. The advice from experienced patients is this: Examine your reasons and try to overcome your reluctance to keep up your social life. Too much time spent in self-imposed isolation isn't good for you. You'll feel better if you continue, as much as possible, your usual contacts with others and stay out in the world.

However, they add, you may encounter some unfamiliar situations. Laugh and the world may be startled. "I remember the first time I went to my club and was having a good laugh with a group of the men and two or three of them gave me very odd looks," recounted one man. "For a minute I couldn't think why. Then I realized they were wondering how a guy with cancer could find something funny. 'Hell,' I said, 'I haven't got cancer of the funny bone.'"

Some people may ask blunt and insensitive questions. "I wish somebody had warned me to expect a few shockers," said a mother. "I might have been braced for them when my son, who was then three, was being treated for leukemia." She remembers being asked if treatment would damage his brain.

Another woman who had a mastectomy recalls being confronted by a casual acquaintance who wanted to know which breast she'd had removed. She fled in tears. Family members report they are asked, "How long did the doctor give her?" by acquaintances inquiring about a relative with cancer. Few doctors today play God and set a time limit for any individual life. Nobody can know how long a person has to live. "If you're not prepared for such questions, it can pull the rug out from under you," said the husband of a patient.

Some questions deserve no reply. Some queries may make you feel people are prying. Said one woman, "I came to see that a reason for people asking questions that appeared to me to be rude curiosity was their own fear of cancer. They were trying to find out from me what it felt like in case they got cancer too." She said it made her feel less irritated by personal questions. But, she added, it didn't make her feel obliged to answer them. She either told her questioner she didn't wish to talk about it or simply ignored the question and changed the subject.

On the credit side, patients say they found some friends turned out to be genuine jewels. They meant it when they offered help and quickly picked up on any suggestions about how they could be useful. In some cases friends helped the patient by giving their support to the family. "When Tom was in hospital I felt totally alone," said one wife. "He had people around him, friends and doctors, but I didn't know a lot of people. We'd moved here quite recently. It made a big difference to me when one of Tom's business friends and his wife took me under their wing. Tom felt better to see me less depressed."

Patients returning to work after treatment has the cancer under control may find fellow workers uneasy with them. It can be disappointing when companionship one has looked forward to enjoying again is strained. Some people found it eased matters if they spoke frankly about their disease the first couple of days so that others realized they need not tiptoe around them, fearful of letting an upsetting comment slip out. Others, who preferred to say nothing, found co-workers soon became comfortable with them again when the patients went about business as usual and behaved as they always had.

Not all patients can return to their former jobs. Some need lighter work or a workplace where there is less risk of infection. They may have to consider retraining or make other plans for alternative employment.

Society is gradually becoming more enlightened about cancer and patients are less likely to find themselves out the door as a result of the disease. But it can still happen. A 46-year-old vice-president of a large company, whose employers asked him to resign says, "I hit an all-time low. It never occurred to me my job would be in jeopardy." He says it took him several months to recognize that the company was wrong to assume he would no longer be able to carry his weight. "My confidence in myself took a bad shaking. I was accepting their views that cancer made me second rate." Now, three years later, he heads a small but growing manufacturing company.

In Canada in future, the Canadian Charter of Rights may provide a defence against job discrimination for people with cancer. In the United States, the Rehabilitation Act of 1973 includes cancer patients among handicapped people and is designed to combat discrimination against them. The cancer patient may not be physically or mentally handicapped yet is considered handicapped because misconceptions about cancer limit employment opportunities.

Although Canadians do not have to worry about catastrophic medical and hospital bills, thanks to Medicare which pays hospital and doctors' bills for everyone, a lengthy period of illness can cut into earnings. In the United States the programme called Medicare covers people of age 65 or older and a second programme called Medicaid provides financial assistance for people with incomes insufficient to pay extensive medical costs. People who work for large corporations frequently have extended sick leave benefits that provide continuing income during the period they are unable to carry on with their jobs. Patients working for small companies or who are self-employed may not be as fortunate. In Canada for those who need financial assistance with expenses related to care, some funds may be available from the Canadian Cancer Society. Inquiries can be made through your local or provincial cancer society. The addresses are listed at the back of this book.

Disability or life insurance may be matters of importance to you. Patients tend to believe that buying such insurance while they are undergoing cancer treatment or following it would be either impossible or prohibitively expensive. That is not necessarily so. Insurance companies are designing premium schedules that reflect the improvements in cancer treatment.

It could be worthwhile seeking information from your insurance company. Usually the medical director of an insurance company decides the specific risk in each case. Detailed documentation may be required from your doctors but you should not be discouraged from seeking insurance for fear it will be refused you.

Eight
When a child has cancer

NOTHING SEEMS MORE unjust than cancer in a child. It is not only life that is threatened but the carefree childhood most of us consider the birthright of every child. We know millions of children in the world, for many reasons, won't be so lucky, but we expect ourselves as parents to raise our children in ways that will provide them with fond memories of their childhood days. Cancer demolishes those expectations.

When your child develops cancer, powerful emotions surge forth that can be overwhelming. Parents need to hold tight to the knowledge that treatments of childhood cancers succeed more often than not. They have tipped the scale in favour of life. Normal life. Nevertheless, as with all cancers, there is no guarantee that any particular child's cancer can be banished once and for all. No doctor can say, even after treatment has brought about a remission, "There. That's fixed. Your child won't be bothered with that again."

At the point when a child's cancer is detected, the instinctive reaction of parents and others is to protect the child they love, yet be aware, with heart-stabbing anguish, that they cannot. Parents hear the diagnosis first in most cases. Some of them say that even five or ten years after the child has been successfully treated, that moment stands out vividly as the most painful experience of their lives.

Often the initial reaction of parents is, "Don't tell the child." It is understandable. Unable to protect the child from the disease, they want at least to protect the child from knowing about it. "We

66

can't bear it and we are adults," said one father. "What would it do to my boy if we told him? He's only eight."

Yet doctors and nurses looking after young patients say a child understands what is happening long before the parents are ready to accept the fact that the child knows. "It is shocking to some people how grown up these children get, how fast," said one doctor.

Generally it is considered best to tell the child as much about the illness as the child's age allows him or her to understand. In the past it was assumed children under the age of ten were too young to be aware of the seriousness of cancer. Now it is recognized that young children may have great fear and anxiety although they may not be able to explain their feelings and may ask no questions.

Children who know their illness is more serious than the common diseases of childhood may be doubly afraid if secrecy has isolated them and nobody seems to understand they are worried and afraid. If children do ask and parents don't answer their questions with honesty, they will sense they are not being levelled with and their trust in their parents may be undermined. A child may think he or she has done something so terrible it can't be spoken aloud and be terrified of being abandoned.

Older children whose parents have not talked with them about their cancer can read unspoken clues and know the truth. But they may pretend ignorance just as they did when they first found out about Santa Claus and realized their parents didn't want them to know. But this time the loneliness is awful. It can come as an immense relief when mother and father are finally able to talk openly about it with them. One study of young patients who had their cancers as children or teen-agers and were questioned following treatment found a high percentage of them felt the diagnosis should be shared with children early.

It takes time for parents to gain a realistic understanding of the disease and the treatment themselves. Parents say they could not retain everything they needed to know with the first telling and needed explanations repeated. "A train was barrelling through my head. I couldn't hear what I was being told," said one mother. A youngster's response to his or her illness will be influenced in large measure by how the parents react. They are, after all, the people who are central to the child's existence. Parents say they knew they had to master their own despair in order to demonstrate genuine optimism and courage to their children.

Some couples found they had first to work out their own differences. Their emotional reactions to the diagnosis were at odds or they disagreed on decisions that had to be made. Even basically sound families found the inordinate amount of stress they were under created tensions they had not anticipated in the marriage. In some cases the mother was spending a great deal of time with the child in hospital and came to consider herself part of the treatment team while the father, feeling lost and uninvolved, had a hard time developing a realistic perspective on the situation.

"We went through a rough time between ourselves," explained one woman. "Larry, my husband, had to be out of town a lot on business. I was trying to keep him filled in on everything. It began to seem we never talked about anything else. Larry was feeling the same way, yet he felt guilty he couldn't be more help to me or our daughter." Their relationship began to suffer, she said. Each felt increasingly neglected and misunderstood by the other. "I think we came perilously close to ruining a perfectly good marriage." She added, "Tell parents to look after themselves as a couple as well as devoting themselves to their child. What would it have been like for our Julie to come out of hospital to a messed-up home?"

A parent may well wonder if it is possible to stand up under the emotional load. There is so much to be dealt with all at one time. They are confronting fear, their own fear and their child's, trying to overcome their anger and guilt, learning about the illness and its ramifications, interpreting what is happening to the child, both to the patient and possibly to other children in the family, seeking to gain insight into each other so they can pull together, and often keeping grandparents or other relatives informed and consoled. "I felt everybody was leaning on us but there was nobody we could lean on," one father said.

Meeting with other parents of children with cancer can be helpful and some hospitals arrange programmes for parents. Many parents say they found the strength to cope because they had to. There was no choice. "You keep going because if you fall over you will desert your child. You can't do that," said one parent.

Leukemia is the most common childhood cancer and its treatment has improved dramatically in recent years. Usually after a week to a month in hospital, the child is able to go home. The disease will be under control although the child continues to have treatment at regular intervals. In most cases it is possible for the child to return to school. The idea may alarm parents who are fearful of letting the youngster out of their sight. They may keep postponing the return. "Overly-protective parents fail to see the value of school to the child," says one specialist. "School is a child's work. It is where he makes friends and learns about the world and how to get along in it."

When children have been away from school for a while, they may shy away from going back to class. They figure they have fallen behind in schoolwork and don't know what to expect from classmates now that they are "different" from other children. Youngsters quickly learn to manipulate parents who are worried about them, say child experts. A child can put on a most convincing act of feeling unwell, only to undergo a remarkable recovery as soon as the school bus has departed or it is too late to attend class that day. One review of school attendance of children with cancer found attendance plummeted the first year after diagnosis, which might be expected, but also that it was still well below average three years later among children free of all signs of diseases.

A lengthy absence from school means friendships fade and life is much less normal than it need be for the child. Parents should master their own anxieties and encourage the child to miss as little school as possible.

Child specialists say it is wise for parents to visit the child's teacher and discuss the situation. Does the teacher have answers to questions the other children may ask? If, for example, the young patient has hair loss will the teacher say something like, "It is because Evan is taking medicine just now, but it will grow back"? Or will the teacher's own fears of cancer throw him or her into a tizzy? If a teacher's understanding of cancer is not all you would wish, you might enlist the aid of the school nurse.

Having a chat with a few of the child's friends can also be a good idea. Children, out of ignorance, can taunt or be cruel but they have a tremendous capacity to support another child if they are given information that allows them to understand. One mother was so afraid her child would be asked by neighbourhood playmates if he was going to die, she couldn't bring herself to allow him freedom to play with them. Her own fear was projected onto her child. Trying to shelter him, she was interfering with his development and his fun.

Brothers and sisters need to know as much about the patient's illness as they are able to comprehend. They may worry about whether they are going to get sick too. They need reassurance this disease is not like the chicken pox they all caught. Sometimes a brother or sister secretly believes the illness is his or her fault. In the heat of a scrap it's not uncommon for a child to wish a sibling didn't exist. Young children often believe they can actually make things happen by wishing. They need to have it made clear that nobody caused the disease and it wasn't their doing no matter what they might have wished.

Other children in the family need their share of attention more than ever at a time when parents and other relatives are expressing so much concern about one child. It may be difficult to find the time and the energy to ensure that the healthy children don't feel neglected and unloved. Grandparents or other relatives can help fill in but the other children still need the attention of their all-important parents. People in a family sometimes expect too much of the other youngsters. Parents may then be appalled when a child takes out his or her frustrations on the patient.

Children can derive bizarre notions about what is happening to the patient in hospital. As early as possible, if circumstances permit, brothers and sisters should be taken to see the patient. Specialists say fantasies may range from imagining the patient is being tortured to thinking special treats are being given. They may be terrified or jealous.

Having a child in hospital may arouse unwarranted doubts in parents too. A parent may start feeling inadequate as a mother or father because others have taken over much of the child's care. Although many hospitals today encourage parents to provide as much of their children's non-medical attention as they can, a hospital is still an unfamiliar environment. Parents may feel uncertain or uncomfortable ministering to their child under the eye of health professionals. If you feel inept, try to remember that despite being an amateur you are the most comforting nurse your child can have.

When parents have to go home, they may experience pangs of uneasiness leaving the child with nurses and doctors they haven't had time to get to know or trust. On the other hand, when parents feel unsure of their own abilities to look after a seriously ill child, they may experience a sense of relief, knowing the child is in the hands of experts.

The child, too, may be distressed when parents leave. Some parents have found it helps comfort a youngster in hospital to be given a tape recording of them reading a story or just talking. Even quite young children can operate a small tape recorder. Nurses have reported their little patients never seem to tire of the repeated message. It is comforting during empty spots in the day when parents cannot be there. Nurses relate that the children typically say things such as, "That's my Mummy," or talk back to the tape, answering it.

Commonly, when parents are able to spend time with the child in hospital, they find they gradually feel better informed and more confident that they will be able to look after the child competently when it is time to return home. Those who have been through the experience say: Don't despair if at first you are flooded with so much information that is new to you that you are in a fog. It has been said we can only learn what we already almost know. In other words, we become knowledgeable bit by bit. Parents say they found they needed to be given information over and over, possibly because they could only absorb a little of it each time. "At times I felt the nurses must think I was really stupid," said one mother.

Sometimes parents feel they are not being given enough information to satisfy them. "It made me angry," said one father. He raged at the doctors. "This is my child but nobody talks to me as if she is."

In a large hospital, a number of people may be taking part in the care of a child. Parents must make sure they know the name of the doctor in charge of the child's case. They have the right to expect that that particular doctor will meet with them at specified times and answer their questions. They also have the right to expect that other specialists treating the child will have kept the doctor in charge of the case fully informed. It is important to have one designated pathway for all medical communication.

If you don't know your child's doctor and have trouble finding him, go to the head of the hospital and ask for assistance. One U.S. study found that 40 per cent of families could not identify the patient's doctor and 46 per cent had never spoken to him or her.

When a child goes into remission it means he or she becomes free of all signs of disease and will probably be able to go home. However, it does not mean treatment is over. Usually therapy to maintain the remission continues for two or three years. During that time the child will undergo repeated tests so that any indication of a return of disease will be spotted quickly. There may still be side-effects of the maintenance treatment. In all, it means family life remains somewhat disrupted.

Sometimes this ongoing encounter with cancer locks parents into traditional roles; mother as a homemaker, father as wage-earner. If a family formerly had two incomes it may mean financial hardships. For a mother who enjoyed working outside the home it can be a sacrifice despite her willingness to put her child's needs ahead of her own. Once again, families may find they are facing adjustments that cause strain. Added to that may be difficulties with the child's behaviour.

Some parents explain that problems arose with the children

because the parents had to re-learn to treat the child as a normal kid. One study found that a number of parents who had discipline difficulties with their children blamed it on the fact that they didn't know what they should reasonably expect of the child in light of the cancer. "I often felt confused about what to let my son get away with," said one mother. "I wasn't sure when to set limits." She realized his treatment sometimes made him irritable and grouchy, yet, she said, she couldn't allow him to take it out on his sister.

In some families, parents overindulge the patient, allowing behaviour they wouldn't accept from a well child. Others buy everything the child desires. They can't do enough, they are so thankful the child is alive. But the message children get is not that they are dearly loved. Rather it is that despite the remission they are sicker than they thought. They know healthy kids aren't treated that way. If they are allowed to tyrannize others in the family, they don't like themselves much either.

The necessary balance isn't simple to attain, parents say. "When the child goes back to school it's hard to know what level of performance you should expect of him," says one family counsellor. "Kids will goof off if they can get away with it and the child with cancer is no different. But he may have missed enough school so he's discouraged and feel he's failing even though he's trying hard."

Parents need a lot of wisdom. The main thing is for them to expect the child will have a future and to help prepare for it as they would have if cancer had never arisen. In any case, simply being accepted, with the cancer neither ignored or dwelt on, is what the child needs most and wants.

Teen-age patients share some of the problems of children with cancer, but they also must cope with the additional conflicts that normally accompany adolescence. It is a period of life when young people are trying to establish independence from parents and to discover who they are as they mature sexually.

Illness may knock the teen-agers' development off course. Abruptly they are back in a state of dependence. Newly won control over their own lives has been yanked away. Their parents may be as anxiously protective of them as they would be if they were small children again. Battles may erupt over everyday matters such as eating and resting. The power struggle between patients and parents can be chaotic.

Physical appearance is critical to the adolescent. Any alteration in looks is far more distressing than it would be to a child or to an older adult. Although people their own age are of prime importance in the development of young people's self-image and esteem, teen-agers may withdraw from them if their appearance has been affected.

Some teen-agers rebel against treatment. Doctors say in a number of cases they have persuaded teen patients to continue treatment only on the ground it will avoid hurting those they love. The won't do it to help themselves.

Their moods may swing from wild optimism to dour depression. They may rage at people who love them or sink into apathy. Parents may find it hard to remember that teen-agers' emotional reactions are in a state of flux even if they are perfectly healthy and that conflict between parent and adolescent child is normal. Parents may not know what the young person is thinking or how to reach out to share feelings. Adolescence is a period when communication between young people and their parents commonly hits rock bottom under the most ordinary circumstances. But cancer adds one more dimension to this already turbulent stage of life and enlarges the distresses.

Specialists say it is usually best to let young people take as much responsibility for themselves as possible. To be blunt, get off their backs. The doctors have found they create better rapport with young patients when they give them, rather than their parents, whatever information there is to relay. Although parents may be present during a visit, the doctor talks directly to the patient, and answers any questions, without allowing a parent to do all the talking for the patient.

Doctors also say it is usually quite reasonable to put the patients' non-medical care into their own hands. Parents may not realize how mature the adolescents can become in the wake of illness. There is probably no need to hound them about rest or diet. Given the opportunity to be recognized as the people responsible for their own well-being, they will handle it well most of the time.

Chances are good a young person will reach adulthood with no psychological scars from having had cancer. In a survey of 142 young adults who had cancer in their teens, it was found 86 had attended college, 76 had married, and 46 had children. Psychological problems attributed to cancer were exceedingly rare among them. Although a group of former patients says they wouldn't want to go through adolescence again with cancer, it did not destroy their lives. Said one man, now 23, "I think the toughest part was trying to keep friendships. Everybody but me seemed to have so much energy. I couldn't keep up and I felt I missed out on a lot." But, he added, "It could have been worse. I'm here. I'm okay. And I just got the job I've been after." He's too busy looking forward to regret the past.

Nine
Self-help programmes

THERE WILL PROBABLY be times when you feel nobody can understand what you are going through. But there are people who know. They've been there earlier or are travelling the same path right now. More than thirty years ago people with cancer began to see that they could bolster each other in ways that no one else could. Bonds between patients can be lifelines for people awash with anxiety.

In most communities, patients of any age and with any kind of cancer may contact others who share their experience. One way is through a programme called CanSurmount. If a patient or physician requests it, a CanSurmount volunteer will visit the patient at home or in hospital. Your local cancer society branch can give you information about contacting CanSurmount or you can find the addresses of national and provincial or state cancer societies at the back of this book.

CanSurmount started in Denver, Colorado in 1973. It spread to Canada, beginning in Calgary, Alberta in 1979. The driving force in bringing CanSurmount to Canada is Esther Robins who subsequently was honoured by the Canadian Medical Association for her contribution to health care. Speaking at a Canadian Cancer Society conference, Mrs. Robins said that until she visited Denver two and half years after her cancer was diagnosed, she had never met anybody alive with lymphoma, the kind of cancer she developed.

"Everybody knew somebody who had died of lymphoma and many people really told me all about it in great depth. But I'd never met anybody who was well," she said. "It was more than a revelation for me. It was really the beginning of the realization that I could come to terms with a life-threatening disease and lead a constructive, valuable kind of life.

"I know," she continued, "that my acceptance of cancer would have come about much more easily and with much less heartache if I'd had someone to talk to when I was first diagnosed."

She explained, "As we all know, life is full of change, divorce is prevalent, people are so mobile, they move from place to place, the family group is not what once it was and I think people don't have the roots they once had.

"This is where CanSurmount comes in. We find people who have no one to turn to, don't know who to talk to and what to do. This is where we come in—as concerned listeners who've been there."

A Toronto man who is a volunteer visitor says, "We can deliver something to another patient that no one else can—a living example of coming to terms with cancer and restructuring a life that has both quality and quantity." However, he adds, "Others can help but they can't do it all for you. Only the patient can find an internal strength to contain the crisis and develop a new philosophy by which to retain a reasonable quality of life."

A psychologist says most patients do find their core of tenacity. "They get up in the morning and pour the coffee even knowing they have cancer," she says.

Yet there are periods when others in the same boat make the rowing less onerous. Group programmes for patients and families prove to be sources of great assistance for many people. Examples of such programmes are Coping with Cancer and Living with Cancer, provided through the Canadian Cancer Society. Health professionals guide discussions at meetings but families learn largely from each other. Seeing how others manage may give one a better perspective on one's own strength and emotions.

People who have joined such groups say they picked up valuable practical tips about everything from dealing with nausea after chemotherapy to fielding questions from outsiders. From the experiences of others, you can choose mechanisms of coping that suit your situation, they say. It is often easier to see in others reactions that are adding to their burdens than to see similar responses in yourself. You may see clearly, for example, that the guilt another person is suffering is totally unwarranted and then realize your own feelings of guilt are equally unfounded.

For women who have had mastectomies, a mastectomy visiting service, sponsored by the Canadian Cancer Society is widely available. In the United States a similar service called Reach to Recovery is sponsored by the American Cancer Society. Your local cancer society can put you in touch.

Volunteers, who themselves have undergone breast surgery, visit patients who have recently undergone operations. When a woman, following the surgery, can identify with a healthy woman who has overcome the same difficulties the patient now faces, it is a much less lonely and frightening experience.

The American programme, Reach to Recovery, started in New York by Mrs. Terese Lasser, was adopted by the American Cancer Society as a national programme in 1969. Since then it has been extended to other regions of the world, to Europe in 1974 where it is now available in more than twenty countries and to Asia in 1983. Each country adapts the programme to its own culture and traditions but the basic goal is the same everywhere. It is to show new patients that women with mastectomies are no different from other women. They work, look after their families, make love and play sports. These women encourage the new patient to realize she can do the same.

Organizations for ostomy and laryngectomy patients who have undergone bowel or throat surgery also have programmes to help patients adjust to physical changes through the example of members who had already done so and still lead satisfying lives. Ostomy patients have artificial openings through which body waste is eliminated. Laryngectomy removes the voice box. Names and addresses of these organizations are listed at the back of this book.

Candlelighters is an organization for parents of young children with cancer which has branches in most states. Other American programmes for people with cancer and their families are I Can

Cope and Make Today Count. See the back of this book for addresses.

While cancer self-help groups play an important role, nobody should invest all their energy in cancer and involvement with other cancer patients. For a time, cancer may override your interest in other subjects and activities. But don't let it take over your whole life. Other aspects of living are necessary diversions from disease.

There are other places or methods that may help you learn to come to grips with your disease. "Respect your mind, respect your body and respect your spirit," says one specialist. "We know what cancer can do to a patient but we don't know yet what a patient can do to his cancer. There may be effects of the interaction of body, mind and spirit in coping with cancer more powerful then we guess."

Many people turn to their religious faith to gain strength and peace of mind. For those with strong faith it can be a bulwark against despair. "Everyone has a spiritual life. Not everyone has a formal religious life," says a clergyman with special experience in ministering to cancer patients. "When the disease of cancer is diagnosed, the human spirit is immediately affected."

While some people who did not previously consider themselves religious may discover a faith within themselves, others feel no urge to seek solace from a divine source. Some people take comfort from the traditions of their church and others want no formal religious package. Yet, say people who offer spiritual counselling in hospitals, most patients have spiritual needs that require attention. "Persons with cancer are undergoing all sorts of emotional, ideological and spiritual challenges," says one.

In some instances, patients believe cancer is divine punishment for their sins and suffer spiritually. "God does not cause cancer to make a person shape up," says one chaplain. Nor, he says, does cancer indicate a person has been abandoned by God as some patients fear. Such people may need more than medical treatment. Each patient must determine individually where to seek assistance for spiritual distress if the need arises. A growing number of members of the clergy have been trained in dealing with the extraordinary impact of cancer. It is probable a chaplain associated with a treatment centre has such expertise. Patient or family may feel this person is someone to whom they can turn if their own minister or priest is too far away or if they do not belong to a church or religious congregation.

If spiritual health can help the body deal with disease, it is a two-way street. Physical activity may reduce mental anguish. You may feel there isn't much you can do for your body right now. It is not as though getting fit will eliminate your cancer. Yet studies show patients who exercise feel less tired. At one hospital it was found that exercise sessions amounting to 45 minutes a week brought a marked drop in anxiety among patients, that anger and hostility were reduced and cheerfulness increased. If your doctor approves, you may find you can help yourself considerably through an exercise programme. The kind of exercise will, of course, depend on your condition and preference. But it may boost your morale to concentrate on putting health into your body instead of waiting for doctors to get disease out.

A quite different way that a number of patients have found to help themselves is by keeping a journal or diary. One woman said she began her journal simply to maintain a personal record of her treatments. But, she said, she soon found she could pour out into the diary feelings she couldn't air in any other way. "It was kind of a purge," she explained. "If I'd said to my husband some of the things I wrote in that notebook, he'd have been dreadfully upset." Furthermore, she said, when she looked back over earlier months she could see the progress she was making in learning to cope. "I feel good about that. I can prove to myself things don't seem as bleak to me now as they did. Maybe I've been able to coach myself to be able to think more positively. Maybe I'm getting better at living with cancer."

You may discover innovative ways of helping yourself that haven't been touched on here. The important thing to know is that there is almost always something you can do. You are not powerless. You, not your doctor, are in charge of healing your mind and your spirit.

Ten
Remission

THE DAY YOU have been longing for arrives at last. Treatment is over. Your cancer has been stopped in its tracks. Wonderful, isn't it? It is. But it may not bring the sense of relief and joy you anticipated. A number of people who reached that milestone say they were surprised at their own mixed feelings. They had visualized the moment when they would shed the label of "patient" and rejoin the ranks of the well so they could get back to normal living.

Yet, they said, they felt a new uprising of anxiety. They were uneasy being on their own, no longer under the constant surveillance of a medical team. One woman described it as "a pushed out of the nest" feeling. She felt scared.

There will be check-ups at regular intervals. Follow-up visits to the treatment centre or doctor will continue for many years. Nobody can tell you your cancer is cured. It may be. But it isn't possible to know at the time treatment ends. It has been said that to ask, "What is a cancer cure?" is the wrong question. The question should be "*When* is a cancer cured?" Most physicians agree a patient can be considered cured if there is no detectable disease five years after treatment. But even then there is no ironclad guarantee it will never return. Some patients say they determined to push their encounter with cancer out of their minds and never think of it again. They could do so much of the time but, they said, you can't really forget having had cancer. Even if you are feeling fine and have no surgical scars to remind you, the uncertainty of cancer remains.

As one human behaviour specialist put it, "The main emotional task of the long-term survivor of cancer is living while feeling vulnerable."

Some patients say that after they settled back into the ordinary family routines and their relatives had stopped treating them like fragile china, there were only certain occasions when fears re-surfaced, choking them. It might be the anniversary of the date of diagnosis that triggered an echo of former terror. Most said that on the day or two before their regular check-ups they went through acute anxiety. What if it has come back? "It may be impossible for your family to imagine what you are feeling," said one young woman. "I would stay with my mother when I came to the city for my tests. She'd been a tower of strength to me while I was going through treatment and we'd become very close. But right before my check I just froze up and couldn't talk to her at all. She couldn't understand why."

When the patient is a child, anniversaries and check-ups commonly put more stress on the parents than on the child. "I'd be tied in knots. I couldn't sleep," said one mother. "I'd tell myself over and over Maria was so well there couldn't have been a recurrence, but...there is always that damn 'but'."

Many people find that ordinary aches and pains they would once have dismissed as nothing serious set off alarm bells in their heads. "When Bill began feeling wretched one day last winter, both of us almost panicked," says a wife. "The flu had been going around his office and he'd picked up the bug. But flu wasn't our first thought. Ordinary things can seem so ominous."

Certain patients said that although they felt confident the original cancer was gone, they worried about developing another cancer as a result of the treatment. It is true that drugs used to treat cancer are also capable of causing cancer. The patients said they knew the benefit of their treatment far outweighed the risk, but fear nagged just the same.

The chance of a second tumour resulting from treatment is relatively small. In women with breast cancer that has spread beyond the breast and who are treated with chemotherapy, a few will have developed a second tumour ten years later. But without the drug therapy, 80 per cent would have died of their original disease.

For some people, cancer sets their lives off in new directions. A U.S. Senator, Paul Tsongas, gave up his political career when he developed lymphoma. Although his doctors told him there was no reason not to seek re-election for another six year term, he chose to spend more time with his wife and three daughters. "Cancer makes you think about other things," the 43-year-old senator told the *New York Times.* "If I'm going to have regrets, let it be on my political career and not on my family."

A top Canadian newspaperman gave up his executive post on a large daily after his wife was treated for cancer and moved to a small town where the two of them could work together producing a little weekly newspaper.

A significant number of patients and families say they became far more aware of moments worth cherishing. One man told an American Cancer Society conference, "Cancer makes it possible to simultaneously fear test results and dying yet enjoy, perhaps to a greater extent, the simple things of life—sunsets, good food, good moments with those you love."

A 41-year-old journalist working for the Detroit *Free Press* who developed cancer of the eye wrote, "Living with this damnable condition for months now, through times of numb, dumb fear and flashing revelation, what I have embraced are simple truths about basic things—family, friends, strength, weakness, stability, irrationality, the randomness of misfortune, the openess of the future, the common currency of life." He said cynics may sneer. "I sneer a bit myself at myself. I would much prefer finding some new way to deal with this, some fresh glib operating perspective on life and lurking death."

Another man whose cancer is chronic and cannot, he knows, be cured, said he had come to accept living without hope of cure. "Cure, after all, is just a promise we will die of something else," he observes.

Some people speak of learning to live each day more fully as "one of the gifts of cancer." They say in exchange for giving up their belief that their tomorrows would stretch to forever, they were granted the understanding that each day is precious. They live each one to the hilt. "With or without cancer, each of us can only live in our todays," says a woman whom cancer has made wise. She doesn't fool herself into thinking a recurrence would be accepted with grace. She knows, if cancer returns, she may find it more staggering than she did the first time. "But I can't let that possibility spoil today," she says.

Eleven
Palliative care

IF EACH OF us could choose how we die, who among us would select dying alone and in pain?

If we could control how we would spend the final weeks or months of our lives, who would not prefer that time to be lived with style—truly alive until we die.

Yet within the last half-century many people were left to face death alone, uncomforted, and to travel a long barren stretch of existence beforehand. Medicine had become so intent on saving lives, it virtually turned its back on patients who were dying despite medical care. Society in general forgot death was a part of life. Many of us considered death rather like an eclipse of the sun—something one did not look at directly.

Dr. Dorothy Ley, Executive Director of the Palliative Care Foundation of Canada has said, "Modern society has become isolated from life and death over the past three to four decades. We have moved from a largely rural to an urban way of life so that we have become isolated from the daily contact with birthing and dying that was so intimate a part of our ancestors' lives. We are continually exposed to abnormal, violent death and have lost contact with normal death—the end to a beginning."

In recent years a concerted movement has blossomed that is gradually providing for the terminally ill the kind of care that restores death to its proper place as a natural climax of life and restores to the dying their proper place among the living until the moment of death.

It is the palliative care movement. Palliative care is what *can* be done when doctors who are focused solely on cure say there is nothing more to be done. Dr. Ley says palliative care has but a single goal. It is to provide in the remaining time left to a patient suffering from a terminal illness, an improved quality of life, by freeing the patient from as much pain as possible and by alleviating the emotional stress on the patient and his family.

The mother of palliative care is Dr. Cicely Saunders, founder of St. Christopher's Hospice in London, England. It was her example that others followed in the modern revival of palliative care. When her hospice was opened in 1967, Dr. Saunders envisioned a kind of care not then commonly available in most hospitals. Usually the dying were forced to undergo extreme aggressive treatment in attempts to postpone death or were given little care at all. Doctors and nurses hurried past their beds to spend their time on more rewarding cases. Dr. Saunders has called the kind of care given at St. Christopher's 'ELC"—efficient loving care. Its goal, she says, is "that no one should reach that desperate place where he could only ask for his life to be ended."

"We tend to put quotes around people who are dying," she says. "They are still the same persons. We must not isolate them behind the barriers of our own embarrassment."

The philosophy of palliative care spread to North America. By the start of 1984, there were 116 palliative care programmes in Canada. Some general hospitals have allotted special units or beds. Some are community programmes that help families look after patients at home with back-up from hospitals in the community. The Palliative Care Foundation of Canada publishes a directory of the programmes. (Addresses for the Palliative Care Foundation of Canada and the U.S. National Hospice Organization are listed at the back of this book.) Programmes are often called "hospices" even though there may not be a free-standing hospice building. For example, the city of Windsor calls its programme Hospice Windsor although care is provided in the community and in a general hospital. Hospice Victoria is located in the Royal Jubilee Hospital in Victoria, British

Columbia, where a number of beds are designated for palliative care. The hospice is run separately from the rest of the hospital and has its own board of directors.

In the United States by 1984 there were some 1800 hospices, many of them organized and operated by volunteer organizations. The first hospice in the United States was opened in 1971 in New Haven, Connecticut, and was patterned on St. Christopher's. In Canada, in 1975, Royal Victoria Hospital in Montreal began a hospice and bereavement programme which was to expand, through McGill University, into a network of services involving three hospitals and teams of home care workers to provide services to patients in their homes. It has been called one of the most successful and comprehensive programmes in North America.

Palliative care is not restricted to cancer patients but they form about 95 per cent of the people being served by most programmes. Cancer does not bring death abruptly in most cases. Many people in society believe that is the aspect of cancer most to be dreaded. Yet many cancer patients who know they are terminally ill say they would not want to be leapt on by death suddenly and unexpectedly. A sudden heart attack, they say, would have given them no time to make preparations and say goodbye nor to savour cherished moments with those they love.

What does being terminally ill mean? It is not a defined period of time. Nobody knows when any individual will die. But it means that no matter what is done, the person's disease will progress until life can no longer inhabit the body. "It is," said one patient "like looking across a lake that has always been shrouded in fog and then one day you can see the horizon."

When groups of cancer patients were asked where they would choose to die, a majority said they would like to die at home where they could spend more time with people they love and be freer to have things they way they like. "Ideally," says one palliative care planner, "the patient should be in an institution only if pain and symptoms cannot be adequately controlled at home, if the family cannot cope, or if the patient and family wish the patient to die in the institution. Otherwise, efforts should be made to return the patient to his home and support him there as long as possible."

"If there is ever anyone who needs love and support, it is the dying patient," says Dr. Ley. "He is losing everything he knows—family, job, status, control of life. Somebody else will take the role he may have played for fifty years. This is the most important thing that happens in life and it is a time when a person needs to feel comfortable within the family."

For some patients, home is the right place to be. Most families will need some help, perhaps from a palliative care programme if there is one in the community, a hospital out-reach programme, home-care programme, or visiting nurse. In some cases, a doctor who is readily available will be the only professional needed because the skills of family, friends and neighbours can be called on. Without being aware of it, they have become a palliative care team.

One elderly patient cared for at home looked forward each day to a chat with a neighbour who stopped by when she walked her dog. The chat brought the patient a little of the outside world and the funny little dog made her laugh. "The neighbour would never have thought of herself as a member of a palliative care team," says Dr. Ley. "But that is what it is all about, keeping a person alive until he is actually dead by using any method at our disposal."

A family that is considering bringing home from hospital a terminally ill patient must take a number of things into account. Is the lay-out of the home adaptable to a full-time patient? If the person will be confined to bed, there will need to be an adjacent bathroom. Will that mean the patient will be isolated on the second floor apart from family activities?

One person, often wife or husband, may provide the bulk of the patient's care. But care may be required around the clock. Are there others who will spell off the prime household nurse to allow for adequate sleep and avoid exhausting that person?

The family should determine what will be needed in the way of equipment, such as hospital bed, wheelchair, and medical supplies. If no family member has the nursing skills needed to keep the patient comfortable, a professional private nurse may be required.

Possibly most important is to ensure pain can be managed at home. Not all terminally ill cancer patients suffer pain, but if a patient does, pain control is crucial. In some cases it takes highly sophisticated pharmacology planning to achieve a balance whereby the patient is alert but pain-free.

One man, caring for his dying wife, found he didn't need an array of helpers as long as a doctor could keep her free of pain. Housework, preparing meals and bedside nursing were tasks he could do himself and they preferred to be alone together in their small house.

Families must be sure that all members are emotionally prepared to have the patient die at home. Unless they have accepted death as inevitable, when the patient does die, they may blame themselves, convinced the patient would still be alive if he or she was in hospital. They may torment themselves, wondering if death was caused by something they did, or didn't, do.

Teen-age children often have the greatest difficulty facing the death of a family member. One 17-year-old youth left home when his dying father returned home. "At first Ted just stayed out of the house a lot avoiding his father," says his mother. "Then one morning he left a note on the kitchen table and he was gone. I was too preoccupied with his father to see how badly Ted was taking things."

Social workers on palliative care teams have, at times, recognized the distress a young family member is feeling and can't handle. They have understood why young people shut themselves off from family love in a desperate bid to escape pain and grief, and have been able to reach out to them. Many families will need help from people with special understanding of the needs of both patient and family as they deal with the grief of impending loss. There are not, as yet, enough palliative care programmes to meet the need. However, a number of hospitals provide help in planning a patient's return home.

You should discuss with your doctor what to do when death

occurs. The doctor will be required to come to the home and declare the patient dead. Before he arrives, close the person's eyes and mouth. Usually the undertaker will look after arrangements for the body to be moved from the home.

The moment of death is rarely one of struggle. If you have never seen anyone die, you may be fearful of what will happen. Usually the patient has been slipping in and out of consciousness and there is no one single dramatic event. Death advances by degrees moving up the body. The feet feel cold before the upper body and the loss of the use of legs occurs before loss of the arms. Breathing may change, with the number of breaths decreasing.

We may tremble when we imagine keeping a last vigil at home with no call-button to summon nurses or doctors to stop life ebbing away. Yet those who have looked after a dying person at home say there can be enormous rewards. "I remember Gerry propped in the bed we'd rigged up in the family room laughing when our two boys bounced in from school excited over some big deal in class," says one widow. "I see him watching the bluejays that came each day to get peanuts I would put on his windowsill and I hear him exclaiming over the colours of tulips in the bulb garden he'd planted the previous fall.

"It wasn't all easy and beautiful. But those are memories I wouldn't have if he hadn't been home. Those are moments he wouldn't have had."

Not all families are capable of looking after a terminally ill person. We have come to believe a hospital, with all its medical wizardry of technology, is essential. When patient and family decide the patient should be in hospital and know there is no possibility of recovery, it is important to talk about the wishes of the patient concerning measures to prolong life. If the patient does not choose to have resuscitation techniques or machines used to keep heart and lungs going it is best if the family and the doctor know that is how the patient feels.

Not too long ago, rigid hospital rules made it likely a patient in hospital would not have the family present when he or she died. But the spreading of the philosophy of palliative care is bringing change into many hospitals even if they do not have special hospice units. Visiting hours are waived so family members can stay steadfastly by the patient's side. It may be possible for relatives to prepare food the patient fancies at an odd hour. Small children or babies may be allowed to visit.

There is also less likelihood that resuscitation teams will pummel the patient's body to drive life back in for a few more days, particularly if it is known that this is against the patient's wishes. In 1984, the Canadian Medical Association, Canadian Nurses Association and Canadian Hospital Association issued a joint statement on terminal illness which said that while palliative care to alleviate mental and physical discomfort should be provided at all times, heroic life-saving measures that prolong dying are not always necessary. The statement said the family should be involved in making the decision. It is often difficult for the family to let a patient go, but death of the personality may already have taken place. The patient will never come out of a coma.

Inflicting heartbeat and respiration with machines on a dying patient against that patient's wishes is coming to be seen as meddlesome medicine. But at the same time, there is growing belief that people are entitled to write the ending of their own story. Dying with dignity to one person may mean gracefully bowing out without a last-ditch fight. To another, dying without the fiercest fight he or she and the doctors can put up is unthinkable. Someone who has never been a quitter isn't about to start now.

In palliative care units, while traditional medical therapy is used to ease physical pain, other kinds of therapy such as music and art are often used to relieve pain of the spirit. Sometimes they enable patients to let out pent-up emotions a patient cannot release in words. Dr. Balfour Mount, director of the McGill Palliative Care Service in Montreal, has reported the profound impact of music therapy on patients with pain and nausea that drugs could not alleviate. Music therapy has also been able to bring relaxation and sleep to patients exhausted by anxiety, he says.

Painting pictures has become almost standard therapy in

children's hospitals. It is a way of letting small patients express fears and feelings they have neither the vocabulary nor the capacity to speak about and can show those caring for the child what is troubling him or her. There isn't usually a need for special units for dying children. "Palliative care for a child is called Mummy," says Dr. Ley. But palliative care services should encompass the bereaved family and may be needed urgently for parents suffering intense grief following the death of their child.

Doctors have observed that is is not uncommon for a parent to feel a sense of peace when a child with cancer who has been in and out of remission over a long period, dies. It is not an unnatural reaction although others in the family may misunderstand and be worried. The parent has actually gone through the various stages of grief since the shock of diagnosis. That is not to say there won't be many days of deep sadness and feelings of emptiness in the months ahead. But doctors are able to reassure parents they are not abnormal if they feel that way.

Traditions of mourning, observed by past generations or by the peoples of some religions and cultures, contain much wisdom in acknowledging that the period of mourning must be continued for a year or more. They are less common today and this may be a mistake. As one experienced hospice physician says, "Care of the bereaved is the other side of the care of the dying. It is the same coin." Some palliative care programmes extend support to family members after the patient's death.

In some communities there are groups such as Bereaved Parents' Associations (see directory at the back of this book) or programmes through which new widows may find the support of other women whose husbands have died. Grief borne alone may, for some people, become an illness in itself. Bereaved people can die of a broken heart.

Twelve
Unorthodox therapy

IT IS ALMOST a sure bet that one way or another you will hear about an off-beat cancer treatment. You will probably be told that it avoids the unpleasant effects imposed by conventional therapy and be told of people for whom it worked after doctors had given up.

Many patients desperately want to believe what they are told is true. The idea that someone, somewhere is able with ease to restore the health of a person with cancer is irresistible. Self-styled healers have been offering tempting plums to cancer patients for a long, long time and they will continue to do so until the riddle of cancer has been solved and society no longer dreads the disease.

There are a variety of reasons why people turn to unorthodox treatments. Some people have extreme fear of—but little faith in—the treatments reputable doctors provide. One survey in Florida found 20 per cent of people who answered a questionnaire felt the treatments for cancer were worse than the disease. They also thought that there had been virtually no progress in treatments for cancer in twenty years. The survey sampled the general population, not patients, and it isn't known if they would change their minds if they developed cancer. But researchers who conducted the study suggest a number of people among that 20 per cent would be vulnerable to sales pitches for non-conventional therapy. Another study in Pennsylvania found that of more than 300 patients at a treatment centre, 13 per cent had used or were continuing to use unorthodox therapy at the same time.

One group of patients who may seek out alternatives are those who have previously been treated with chemotherapy or radiation but who have had a recurrence. They may be disillusioned and discouraged that treatment failed to keep their disease at bay and believe it has no value, or they may have found the first treatment experience so distressing they are unwilling to undergo it again.

Some patients may have been given so little expectation of a good response to treatment that they are willing to try anything else. "What have I got to lose?" they ask.

There is a segment of society that mistrusts the medical profession, possibly because of an unfortunate past experience or perhaps because they resent the power and prestige they believe is held by the medical profession's "monopoly". Among them are some who claim doctors know a cure for cancer but keep it secret to protect their pocket books. They claim cancer is a big money-maker for doctors, cancer researchers and cancer organizations which they are not prepared to let slip from their grasp. "My God," says one physician, "can people really believe we'd let our own wives, children, parents and even ourselves die of cancer if we knew a cure?" Yet you may hear or read that the medical profession crucifies anybody who puts forward a "real" remedy for cancer. Drug companies and governments are also accused of being in on the conspiracy to protect huge profits being made out of cancer.

How do doctors refute such accusations? Dr. Peter Morgan, scientific editor of the Canadian Medical Association Journal, has proposed doctors take legal action against their accusers. "Such accusations are libellous," he says. However, Dr. Morgan says lay people may get the impression doctors withhold information about medical advances because medical science requires a process known as "peer review." Ethically doctors are required to present their research to other medical scientists (their peers or equals) who are capable of judging the value and validity of the research findings before the news is released to the public. The purpose is to protect patients who cannot be expected to have the knowledge necessary to assess a so-called medical breakthrough. Sometimes a discovery does not hold up under peer scrutiny and the researcher must go back to the drawing board. The process forces medicine to move slowly and cautiously but it prevents patients from being prematurely subjected to treatments that turn out to be useless.

If you hear rumours of a "breakthrough" that raise your hopes high, but you seem to run into a stone wall when you try to track it down, you can be sure it is not because of any medical profession conspiracy to keep a cancer cure secret. It is because the so-called breakthrough has not turned out to be one at all.

Some people who have consulted their physicians about an unorthodox treatment they have heard about have not been satisfied by the doctors' arguments against the treatment. It is understandable to most of us that doctors will do everything in their power to stop a patient from turning to an unscientific mode of therapy when there is every indication conventional therapy can save the patient's life. It makes doctors angry to see patients wasting their savings or putting the family in debt to chase quack remedies the doctor knows to be worthless.

Yet families may not be convinced when, as is often the case, doctors treating cancer patients can make no promises about the outcome of the treatments they themselves provide. At such times, to be scolded for wasting family funds cuts little ice. Few families are prepared to put money ahead of the patient's health.

Even people who have great confidence in their doctors may be seduced by the promotions and promises of those who tout unorthodox treatments. Glowing testimonials from people who have used them are part of the lure. Doctors are not convinced by such testimonials. They know that although the people giving the testimonials may be quite sincere, they may also be mistaken in believing the unorthodox treatment was the cause of their recovery.

Take, for example, the case of one woman with breast cancer who is convinced a herbal remedy cured her. She had had surgery to remove the lump and her doctors had suggested she also have chemotherapy in case there had been any spread of the cancer.

A cancer tumour sometimes sheds cells that travel in the body and sometimes does not. Those cells cannot be detected unless they start up a new tumour.

The woman refused chemotherapy, choosing to take a herbal medicine instead. She has had no recurrence and she is sure the herbal medicine cured her. It is likely, in her case, there was no spread of cancer. The surgery alone cured her disease and she would be free of cancer whether or not she had taken the herbal medicine. Her case is not proof the herbs worked. On the other hand, it doesn't prove the herbal medicine failed to work. It simply tells doctors nothing. They would want much more solid evidence that the herbs have any effect before they could recommend them to other patients.

In other instances, people have enthusiastically credited quack nostrums when, in fact, they have also had conventional treatment known to cure most people with the same kinds of cancer. A case in point is the wife of comedian Red Buttons who was cured of tongue cancer. She had had radiation, which usually works well against this kind of cancer, and she had also taken Laetrile. Both the comedian and his wife publicly endorsed Laetrile giving it exclusive credit for her recovery. It is far more probable that radiation did the trick, as it has for many similar patients who did not take Laetrile.

You have probably heard of Laetrile. In the 1970s debates over its use by cancer patients made it almost a household word in North America. An estimated 70,000 to 100,000 people were taking it, believing it could both treat cancer and prevent it. Laetrile has been called "the most successful quackery in the history of medicine."

Possibly the most famous North American to try treatment with Laetrile was movie actor Steve McQueen who in 1980 was a patient at a Mexican clinic where he was given the substance as part of a treatment regime that also involved coffee enemas and a special diet. The actor had a rare kind of lung cancer that was probably caused by exposure to asbestos earlier in his life when he worked aboard ship. Although, for a short time, there were reports from Mexico that the well-known patient was improving, he died of his disease within a few weeks.

Laetrile, also known as amygdalin and Vitamin B 17 (although it is not a vitamin) was discovered in the 1920s by a California physician, Ernest Krebs, while he was experimenting with flavourings for bootleg whisky. It is made from apricot pits. His son, Dr. Ernest Krebs Jr., claimed to have purified it and coined the name Laetrile in 1952.

In the 1950s, you may recall, the medical profession had little to offer cancer patients other than surgery. Chemotherapy was in its infancy and high-energy radiation was brand new. Inevitably, patients were looking elsewhere for help.

Medical scientists could find no evidence that Laetrile had any value in curbing cancer. The governments of Canada and the United States never gave Laetrile the status of a legal drug.

In Canada, where one of its leading proponents was Andrew McNaughton, son of a former commanding officer of the Canadian Armed Forces, Laetrile was made and distributed by the McNaughton Foundation. But in 1964, the Foundation was prosecuted for marketing Laetrile illegally and Andrew McNaughton moved his operation to California. When that too was shut down, he set up shop in Mexico.

Sales of Laetrile in Canada have remained illegal and many Canadians who sought Laetrile treatment made expensive treks to Mexico or West Germany. In the 1960s Laetrile seemed to be fading gradually from the scene. But in the 1970s in the United States, there was a new surge of support for the apricot pit medicine. It began with the arrest in 1972 of a California physician, John Richardson, who operated a cancer clinic where he used Laetrile in violation of state laws.

Some members of the ultra-right John Birch Society took up Dr. Richardson's cause, arguing that patients should have freedom of choice and putting the weight of the society's publicity and political machinery behind Laetrile promotion. A president of the Birchers, who distributed Laetrile, was estimated, in 1976, to be taking in $150,000 to $200,000 a month in sales.

Public pressure on the federal government in response to the newly aroused interest in Laetrile, forced the U.S. National Cancer Institute to undertake new studies. In the first study the NCI asked patients or doctors to tell it of cases in which Laetrile had worked. The researchers had expected at least two to three hundred cases. They got 93, but medical records documenting the person actually had cancer were available for only 67 people. A panel of twelve cancer specialists judged the cases which were mixed with an equal number of conventionally-treated cases. The judges did not know which patients had taken Laetrile. They decided on the basis of evidence of the state of each patient's cancer before and after treatment. Six of the patients in whom they found there had been improvement had taken Laetrile. However, it could not be shown for certain that nothing other than Laetrile had contributed to the improvement.

A second study, to treat about 150 to 200 patients with Laetrile who volunteered to take part in the test began in 1978. This study, called a clinical trial, investigated Laetrile in the same scientific way any new drug is tested. Laetrile was used by the patients in conjunction with what Laetrile proponents call a programme of total metabolic therapy which includes a vegetarian diet, supplemental vitamins and enzymes and minerals.

When the study was completed in April 1981, the National Cancer Institute reported Laetrile was not effective in treating cancer. Of 178 who took part, 152 patients had died, surviving no longer than would have been expected had they been given no treatment at all.

Laetrile is six per cent cyanide by weight, i.e. one gram contains sixty milligrams of cyanide. Laetrile does not pose a threat if it is injected because it is not broken down and the cyanide is not released. As one doctor says, it simply produces "very expensive urine" as it is excreted by the body. However if it is taken by mouth, the cyanide can be released if certain foods such as almonds, lettuce, celery, peaches or bean sprouts are eaten at the same time. These foods and some others contain chemicals that, mixed with Laetrile, cause the poison to be emitted.

In fact, when Laetrile was first sold it was promoted as a poison to cancer cells. Later, with public interest in health foods and vitamins rising, it was relabelled Vitamin B 17. Dr. Ernest Krebs, Jr. claimed cancer is a vitamin deficiency and that Vitamin B 17 was the missing vitamin. Scientists say Laetrile is nothing like a vitamin.

It is fair to assume that with the NCI's study the heyday of Laetrile is over. But there are still groups that defend and promote it. You could be urged to try it.

Another unorthodox treatment that has been around for a long time in Canada is called Essiac. In 1922, an Ontario nurse, Renée Caisse, was given by Canadian Indians a recipe for a herbal medicine that tribes has used against cancer. She called it Essiac, her name spelled backwards. For more than fifty years Nurse Caisse kept her recipe secret and personally treated hundreds of cancer patients, many of whom swore by her treatment as a method that eased their discomfort even if it did not cure them all. In 1977, she revealed the recipe to the Respirin Corporation Ltd. of Toronto. The medicine was made of four wild herbs and taken with a glass of warm water at bedtime.

A five-year clinical trial, authorized by the Canadian federal health ministry, which ended in 1983 showed no particular benefits from the medicine. Patients who took part in the study may continue to get Essiac if they wish but it is no longer authorized as an investigational new drug that may be prescribed for new patients. However, the drug owner, Respirin Corporation, wants to have another test and the Canadian Cancer Society has said that might be worthwhile. There is some indication that the first test was not up to recognized scientific standards. But the federal government is not eager. It says the Respirin Corporation was given every opportunity to demonstrate Essiac's effectiveness but failed to produce any evidence.

In recent years controversy swirled around a treatment devised by a Texas physician, Dr. Stanislaw Burzynski, who claimed peptides found in urine could control the growth of cells. He called his drugs made with peptides Antineoplastons. A number of Canadian patients had gone to Dr. Burzynski's clinic in Houston, but the case of a young Ontario woman brought the treatment widespread public attention. Stephanie Kusan, then age 20, had been unsuccessfully treated in Toronto for a rare tumour in the cheek-bone, and began undergoing treatment in Texas. She and her family wholeheartedly believed it was helping her but the costs forced the family to mortgage their home, seek public donations and ask for government help to pay bills that totalled $75,000 by the time she died in 1984.

Dr. Burzynski was born and educated in Poland, emigrating to the United States about 1970. He was, for a time, an assistant professor of medicine at Baylor College of Medicine in Houston. But, convinced his research was being blocked by the medical establishment, he struck out on his own, establishing his clinic in 1977 and making his own Antineoplastons from human urine. When the supply of urine obtained from a prison was temporarily unavailable to him, he said he had been able to produce the peptides synthetically. By 1982, he had constructed an elaborate, automated, space-age factory to produce Antineoplastons.

Dr. Burzynski did not follow the accepted scientific method of testing his products on animals and submitting data to the U.S. Food and Drug Administration in order to get approval to investigate the use of Antineoplastons in people. The procedure is required for new drugs, but the doctor claimed extracts from human urine worked only in humans and that animal testing would be pointless.

With no evidence that the substances were safe or effective, the FDA put a temporary halt on the treatment of new patients and the American Cancer Society issued a statement strongly urging individuals with cancer not to participate in treatment with Antineoplastons.

Some Canadians who travelled to Houston claimed they had been helped or cured. However, when as a result of the request by the Kusan family that the government pay their medical costs two cancer specialists were assigned by the Ontario government to investigate, they judged Antineoplastons worthless. The two Toronto specialists visited the Houston clinic in the fall of 1982 and asked Dr. Burzynski to show them documentation of his most successful cases. They reviewed twenty cases he selected and found no evidence any of the patients had benefited from Antineoplastons.

Of four patients whom Dr. Burzynski said had achieved complete remissions, the Canadian doctors found three had died of recurrences. The fourth, who had a bladder tumour removed by biopsy at the time of diagnosis, was alive but the Canadians believed the biopsy had removed the whole tumour, curing him.

Furthermore, the Toronto doctors were alarmed that Dr. Burzynski supplied Antineoplastons to Canadian patients to be administered by themselves through catheters. Such catheters (fine tubing) used by lay people were likely to become infected. The doctors said two Ontario patients developed bloodstream infections (septicemia) after returning from Texas and one of them died of septicemia. The Ontario government refused to pay medical costs for Canadians treated by Dr. Burzynski.

In 1982, Dr. Burzynski charged $180 a day for Antineoplastons treatment, plus other charges that brought the cost of treatment to about $4,000 a month. He said only about one in ten patients paid the whole fee. The clinic also raised funds by seeking donations from corporations and individuals. From an office at the back of the clinic, a small separate company operated a well-oiled publicity machine geared to harvesting donations.

The Canadian federal government, open-mindedly, had been prepared to consider allowing clinical trials of Antineoplastons in Canada where Canadian doctors would be permitted to use and investigate them. However, Canadian regulations relating to the establishment of a clinical trial were not met by Dr. Burzynski and the trial did not take place. Dr. Burzynski has been unwilling to divulge the chemical composition of the peptides and the medicines he calls Antineoplastons.

Dr. Burzynski is not the first physician to claim cancer can be treated with urine products. More than thirty years ago in Toronto, Dr. Phillip Glover treated patients with extracts of horse urine. Like Dr. Burzynski, Dr. Glover would not reveal the ingredients of his medicine nor follow the acceptable scientific pathway to testing.

Diets and vitamins have also formed the basis for a variety of cancer treatments over the years and there has been a recent revival of interest. It came about, in part, through the claims of Nobel prize-winner Dr. Linus Pauling that massive doses of Vitamin C have cancer-defeating powers as treatment and prevention.

Dr. Pauling says a person with cancer should, as early as possible in the course of the disease, begin taking two hundred times the amount of Vitamin C that is ordinarily considered necessary, and take it for life. That would be ten grams a day. He has written a book about cancer and Vitamin C and research is conducted at the Pauling Institute in California.

However, other scientists have been unable to confirm his findings. A group of researchers at the Mayo Clinic, Rochester, Minnesota, who tested ten grams of Vitamin C per day in 150 patients, comparing it with a placebo (a look-alike sugar pill), found no useful effect. The patients in the study had advanced cancer and were not candidates for other conventional treatment. In both the group of patients given the vitamin and in the group given the placebo, about six in ten reported they felt improvement but doctors found no appreciable change in the state of their disease. Four in ten of patients who got the real vitamin experienced nausea and vomiting. Dr. Pauling does not believe Vitamin C has been given a satisfactory scientific investigation and remains convinced of its benefits.

Much research is underway in many centres into the usefulness of vitamins, including Vitamins C, A and E, to combat cancer. Results, so far, have been conflicting and the ultimate answer is not in. But generally doctors recommend that patients, like everyone else, are better served by diets that include a good supply of vitamins from a variety of natural foods, such as fresh fruits and vegetables, than by taking megadoses of vitamin supplements. An excess of some vitamins is toxic and dangerous.

It may be fair to say that in the past doctors were unduly suspicious of promoters of nutritional treatment for cancer patients. Often patients who elected to forego conventional treatment in favour of one diet or another could not accept the idea that the cause of their cancer could not be identified. They preferred to believe that things they could understand, like diet, could cause and cure cancer.

The medical profession has come to recognize that nutrition may have a worthwhile role in cancer therapy. However, few doctors would consider diet or vitamins alone to be adequate treatment for cancer. Some unorthodox nutritional therapy is a danger because its proponents urge patients to reject conventional therapy, claiming that the patient's body must be purged of all toxins and poisons, particularly cancer drugs.

Extravagant claims have been made for fasting in the publications of some so-called natural health organizations. Not uncommon are descriptions of patients with tumours the size of melons that shrank to walnut-size after a fifty-day fast, or other incredible claims. Some publications of this ilk describe raw food vegetarian diets as cures or advertise food supplements such as selenium or zinc as products to both cure cancer and stop aging.

You might wonder what it is that people who promote fasting could be selling. Primarily, the products are books and magazines and the service of non-medical practitioners, as well as memberships in so-called natural hygiene or health organizations that offer to help patients learn to starve out tumours.

The problem with these claims is that tumours compete with normal tissue for nutrients. Because they are growing rapidly, tumours may be quicker to scoop up whatever is available and if the supply is short, normal tissue is deprived rather than cancer tissue. Researchers are investigating ways of selectively withholding from tumour cells essential amino acids and vitamins. But as yet there is no slick way to do that. Patients undergoing treatment need good nutrition to enable the body to make repairs and they generally get better responses to treatment if they are properly nourished.

Advocates of maverick cancer treatments are quick to jump on bandwagons and steer them in directions to suit themselves. Currently they are capitalizing on public interest in fitness. They are also quick to snap up reputable scientific finds to use for their own purposes. For example, scientists are investigating a substance called interferon, produced in the body to fight virus infections. Fake interferon tablets, selling for a dollar apiece, soon appeared on the market as news of interferon research reached the public. Similarly, when experimental treatments of killing cancer cells with heat were reported "hyperthermia" shops cropped up where some unethical practitioners injured or burned people with heat treatment. In some areas of the United States lawsuits were launched against a number of these practitioners who had burned or virtually boiled cancer patients.

People who provide unorthodox therapy commonly purport to have a doctorate in some kind of health care. Some of them actually do have an M.D. or Ph.D. degree and are well-educated scientists. Others are fringe practitioners or have bought their diplomas from unethical or non-existent "colleges." They skirt the law by labelling themselves Ms.D. (Doctor of Metaphysics) or Ph.N. (Philosopher of Naturopathy), according to the American Cancer Society.

You may realize you should be wary of those who do not hold a licence to practise medicine. But what about scientists who have legitimate degrees? How do you tell if they are suspect? Cancer societies have compiled a number of characteristics common among these doctors. Typically they practise apart from medical schools, comprehensive cancer treatment centres or other scientific institutions where their work would be scrutinized by colleagues. They are often at odds with organized medicine and claim it has hindered their efforts. If you ask why the medical profession does not accept their therapy, they tend to compare themselves with great physicians from earlier eras, such as Louis Pasteur, whose innovative work brought him scorn from the medical establishment of the day.

Their medical records are often lacking or skimpy, making it virtually impossible for the value of their treatment to be judged by other doctors. If scientific evaluation of their therapy is made by other reputable scientists and found wanting, they refuse to accept the results, claiming the study was flawed. Frequently they keep their method of treatment secret so that it is available to patients only from them. They may "treat" patients already successfully treated by conventional therapy, yet claim credit for the cure. Some use conventional drugs in combination with their own product but claim favourable effects came only from the latter.

Testimonials from patients who believed they were helped or from their families are an earmark of off-beat practitioners. Often the testimonials are from well-known people, entertainers or politicians who may be sincere but are uninformed or misled. Yul Brynner, who has been starring in the theatrical production, *The King and I* since his lung cancer was diagnosed in September 1983, went to West Germany for a controversial treatment with carrot juice and natural foods in the spring of 1984. While the 66-year-old actor has not actively promoted the German doctor's diet, claims have been made that it has beaten his cancer. However, in 1983 Brynner received radiation therapy for seven and a half weeks during which he did not miss a single performance. At the time his response to treatment was called "spectacular" because when it began it was assumed he had only a few months to live. The actor has been consistently optimistic and says, "Each day is a new day and it is the beginning of the first day of my life."

While in the actor's case, there was no doubt he had cancer, frequently there is no documentation to prove that people who have claimed to be cured by an unorthodox method ever had cancer. Women who have had benign cysts, which are not cancer, removed from their breasts, have believed they were saved from the distress of a mastectomy by some dubious therapy they subsequently took.

In Canada any treatment given by a medical doctor that is not a treatment paid for by Medicare warrants your suspicion. You would be wise to find out more about the treatment and the doctor before submitting to it. If it is an experimental treatment, not yet covered by Medicare because it is still under investigation, there will be no cost to you, and the treatment must have the approval of the hospital or medical school ethics committee or be approved as an investigational new drug by the federal government's health protection branch.

Most tragic are instances in which people have chosen to try treatment provided by an unscrupulous quack before consulting conventional cancer specialists then find, too late, their cancer could have been successfully treated by accepted methods.

Not all unorthodox cancer therapies are quackery or fraud. Some methods that are outside the mainstream of cancer treatments and are considered unproven treatments may be useful to certain patients when they are used in conjunction with regular therapy. One example is a process known as imaging or visual imagery, pioneered in the 1960s by Dr. Carl Simonton, a radiation oncologist in Fort Worth, Texas, and by Stephanie Matthews-Simonton, a psychotherapist.

Patients were taught to visualize in the mind's eye the battle going on within their bodies between their white cells in the immune system and cancer cells. The white cells were the heroes and cancer cells weak and confused creatures. Treatment zapped the tumour like a hail of bullets. Some patients saw their white cells as White Knights, thundering into combat with lances gleaming. It is not suggested that imagery cures cancer by itself, but a few studies have shown that some people who could visualize their warrior cells winning every skirmish had fewer side-effects from treatment and some lived longer than had been expected. Studies done by psychologists have found that people, who of their own accord without coaching saw their white cells as strong and large, Vikings or piranhas, for example, frequently improved while those who saw cancer cells as formidable creatures or clinging like leeches, tended to do less well.

Although some surgeons and physicians concede imaging may have some value, the bulk of the medical profession has remained sceptical. Patients must genuinely believe in the images. It may be that how they visualize their own internal battles is a reflection of their will to live and the extent of their determination to win over cancer. Few doctors would say a patient's will to live is an unimportant factor and many recovered patients are positive that because they were convinced they would overcome cancer, they did.

It is also possible there is a placebo effect. It is a phenomenon well known to doctors. It works this way: when patients are given substances or treatments that they firmly believe will help them, they may improve even if what they were given was really a harmless dummy pill with no medical ingredients. There is growing evidence that a placebo can actually change body chemistry. For example, research has shown that in the brains of people given a placebo to kill pain, brain chemicals, called endorphins, which are neutral pain killers built into the body, respond. The mind, thinking it has received a pain-killing drug, causes the body to act as though it really had. As one doctor says, "The brain can write and fill prescriptions."

Placebos cannot cure cancer. But if they give patients confidence their cancer will be overcome, they may have an impact. A British study of 69 breast cancer patients, reported in the medical journal *The Lancet,* found that those women with a fighting spirit and positive expectations were far more likely to improve than those who accepted their disease with resignation or feelings of hopelessness.

Some patients who by their basic nature cannot sit back passively during treatment but must get into the fray personally, may want to try a method such as imagery if their doctors approve. It does not interfere with regular treatment. Its one hazard is that because it gives patients a feeling of responsibility in the fight against their disease, they may also feel responsible if cancer recurs, slumping into a trough of self-blame. The American Cancer Society lists the Simonton therapy as an unproven method of cancer management it does not recommend for current use.

Among other methods on the Cancer Society's "unproven" list is a Greek cancer treatment that has been promoted in North America by some travel agents. It was devised by a physician in an Athens clinic who kept his medicine a mystery, although he was reported to be willing to sell the formula for seven million dollars. An American doctor who posed as a patient and subjected himself to the treatment brought back to the United States a sample of the medicine for analysis. It was found to be nicotinic acid (niacin) which is part of the Vitamin B family.

You are not likely to hear of all the methods on the Cancer Society's list. A number have disappeared from the marketplace, although there is always a possibility they will resurface. Quack remedies have a tendency to be recycled.

One substance on the list that is still around is the commercial solvent DMSO, dimethyl sulfoxide. It has had more publicity as a remedy for sprains and strains suffered by athletes or for arthritis than for cancer. It is not licensed for use in these conditions but is for a limited number of rare diseases.

DMSO is an enigma. It can travel through the skin and into tissue. It has been controversial since the discovery in the 1960s that it had a medical potential. Dr. Stanley Jacob, a surgeon at the University of Oregon, Portland, pioneered research. The difficulty with DMSO is that it cannot really be controlled by drug laws. People can buy it in industrial strength as a paint-stripper or get it from veterinarians to treat horses or other injured animals. To have a little-understood and unusual drug on the loose in hardware stores and animal clinics scared drug authorities who did their best to ban it.

Dr. Jacob has never proposed that DMSO *per se* could treat cancer. But because it can carry other chemicals along with it into the body, it was suggested it might become a vehicle for administering cancer drugs into tumours. It also received publicity as a pain killer for cancer patients when a former Indiana governor, Dr. Otis Brown, told the American Medical Association he had used veterinarian DMSO to relieve the pain suffered by his wife who was dying of bone cancer.

Quack practitioners, as is their wont, latched onto the public awareness of DMSO and promoted it as treatment for superficial skin tumours. Some injected it as treatment for bladder cancer, although it is not known whether the injections they gave actually contained DMSO.

But in the 1970s reputable British scientists discovered DMSO could protect animal tissue and cells from damage caused by freezing. It began to be used widely in research labs where scientists store tissue samples in deep freezes. In one laboratory where scientists had frozen mouse leukemia cells, it was found that when the cells were thawed, they had changed into near normal cells. Cancer cells are immature cells, stuck at the reproducing stage of the cell cycle. Apparently DMSO had triggered cell maturation.

Since then, in further studies, scientists have found that other solvents, related to DMSO, could cause maturation of human cancer cells in the test tube. One of these substances, called N-methylformanide, made human tumour cells being grown on mice, mature. (Scientists use human tumours, grafted onto mice as a way to study a growing human tumour.)

Currently, this chemical cousin of DMSO is under scientific investigation to determine if it could possibly be of use in humans. If it can make cancer cells become more normal, it might open the door to a new kind of treatment that reforms cancer cells instead of killing them. But it will be a long time before it is known whether reformed cancer cells will stay reformed or slip back into their old ways.

This tantalizing discovery may spur a new flurry of promotions of quack treatment with DMSO. No ethical practitioners use DMSO in the treatment of cancer. Its only use in patients is in some radiation treatment centres where it is used in an attempt to protect normal tissue from radiation damage. There is some evidence that as well as protecting tissue that is frozen, it can also protect against radiation damage. At this time, any other DMSO cancer therapy is outside the stream of acceptable medical treatment.

The only thing known to cure cancer that isn't brought about by conventional treatment is the miracle of spontaneous remission. For no apparent reason, a cancer disappears. It happens only rarely, occurring in fewer than one per cent of cases. It seems to happen most often in cases of malignant melanoma, but even then it is infrequent.

Because spontaneous remission has been observed to be associated sometimes with an infection or fever, it is thought possible that the immune system has been stirred into greater activity by the infection and in the process attacks tumour cells. Yet all sorts of agents that stimulate the immune system have been tried with little success. Spontaneous remission remains a baffling wonder.

Any unscientific treatment you have heard about that you think is worth a try should be discussed with your doctor. A lot of patients do not want to admit to their physicians that they intend to follow some unorthodox regime. They are afraid the doctor will scold them or banish them from his or her care.

Yet it is only sensible to learn as much as you can about any therapy you intend to try and that includes learning any reasons why your doctor disapproves of it. The decision is still in your hands, but what you don't know *can* hurt you. Be informed before you decide.

1984 ESTIMATES

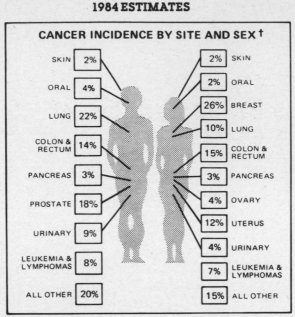

CANCER INCIDENCE BY SITE AND SEX †

SKIN	2%		2%	SKIN
ORAL	4%		2%	ORAL
			26%	BREAST
LUNG	22%		10%	LUNG
COLON & RECTUM	14%		15%	COLON & RECTUM
PANCREAS	3%		3%	PANCREAS
			4%	OVARY
PROSTATE	18%		12%	UTERUS
URINARY	9%		4%	URINARY
LEUKEMIA & LYMPHOMAS	8%		7%	LEUKEMIA & LYMPHOMAS
ALL OTHER	20%		15%	ALL OTHER

† Excluding non-melanoma skin cancer and carcinoma in situ.

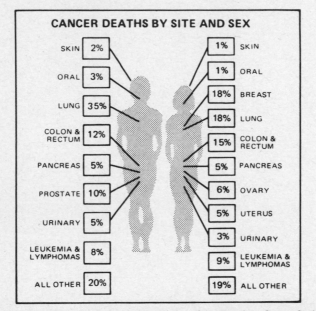

CANCER DEATHS BY SITE AND SEX

SKIN	2%		1%	SKIN
ORAL	3%		1%	ORAL
			18%	BREAST
LUNG	35%		18%	LUNG
COLON & RECTUM	12%		15%	COLON & RECTUM
PANCREAS	5%		5%	PANCREAS
			6%	OVARY
PROSTATE	10%		5%	UTERUS
URINARY	5%		3%	URINARY
LEUKEMIA & LYMPHOMAS	8%		9%	LEUKEMIA & LYMPHOMAS
ALL OTHER	20%		19%	ALL OTHER

Illustration reproduced with the kind permission of the American Cancer Society.

PART TWO
The Scientific Side of Cancer

Thirteen
How cancer is detected

DIAGNOSTIC PROCEDURES

IT GOES WITHOUT saying that none of us want to learn we have cancer. Yet, if there is a possibility a tumour is growing somewhere in our bodies, the sooner it is diagnosed the better the outcome of treatment may be. Most of us are aware that early diagnosis is important. According to a Canadian Cancer Society survey, almost nine in ten of those interviewed believed prompt treatment greatly improved the chances of defeating cancer.

Nevertheless, some people who have reason to think they might have cancer do not seek medical attention right away. They may persuade themselves their suspicions are foolish and the symptoms will probably go away or they may be afraid to find out the truth. The Cancer Society survey found that among 2,000 patients only 63 per cent had made prompt appointments with their doctors when they suspected they had cancer.

If you suspect you or someone close to you may have cancer, please let it be clearly understood a book *cannot* tell you. Only doctors, after making thorough investigations, can make the diagnosis. This section of the book is designed only to give you some understanding of the symptoms that might lead your doctor to order investigative tests and of various tests and equipment used in making the diagnosis.

From Cancer Society educational programmes or posters you

may already know some of the signals that warrant your doctor's immediate attention.

The warning signs include:

A sore that does not heal.

A lump in the breast or anywhere else.

Changes in bowel or bladder habits.

Unusual bleeding or discharge.

Difficulty in swallowing, or persistent cough or hoarseness.

Obvious changes in a mole.

Any unexplained change in your normal state of health.

People who need to undergo investigation for cancer are not always aware of it; sometimes a family doctor is the first to suspect cancer when the patient goes for a routine check-up or for some unrelated complaint. For instance, a doctor might find a small lump in a woman's breast that she had not previously noticed or suspect that a patient's long lasting constipation could be a tumour obstructing the bowel.

If your physician's suspicions are aroused, you may be advised to have certain tests and be referred to medical specialists to undergo investigation. The kind of specialist will depend on the symptoms. In general, cancer is diagnosed by looking into the body by means of x-rays, scans and scopes and by taking samples, called biopsies, of body fluid or tissue. Cells in the sample are examined under a microscope by pathologists. Magnified many times, cancer cells usually look quite different from normal cells. As one doctor describes it: "If you see cells that should look like oranges, but they're the size of grapefruits and shrivelled like prunes, you know you are looking at cancer cells."

Virtually any symptom that could make a doctor suspect cancer can be a symptom of some other ailment. Until the doctor has information about the growth and the kind of cells that form it, it is impossible to tell for certain if you have a cancer.

Usually, the first step is to have you undergo an examination involving a diagnostic machine or piece of equipment that lets doctors see a picture or image of the tumour. On the next pages, the most commonly used types of equipment—and how they work—are described. To read about a diagnostic procedure that your doctor has ordered for you, refer to the Contents page at the front of this book. If you know what to expect, you will feel less worried. Some medical machinery looks huge and formidable yet it is quite painless. Advances in diagnostic technology have reduced enormously the need for exploratory surgery.

X-rays

Conventional x-ray equipment is likely familiar to you. Most of us have had a chest x-ray at some time. The x-ray camera is usually operated by a radiology technician and the film is viewed and interpreted by a medical specialist called a radiologist.

An x-ray machine takes a two dimensional picture. Some parts of the body, such as bones, absorb more x-rays than other tissue because they are denser. Shadows of dense tissue show up on the film. Tumours are often also more dense than surrounding tissue and so can be seen on the film.

Mammography

Mammography is an x-ray examination of the breast that shows lumps in soft tissue. The smallest lump that can be felt with the hand is just under one centimetre, or about the size of a small pea, but even smaller ones are revealed on a mammogram. The mammogram cannot show with certainty whether or not a tumour is benign (not cancer) or malignant (cancer). However, it may provide a clue because benign tumours typically have sharp clearly-defined edges while cancer tumours, with their unruly growth, do not.

The latest mammography equipment gives very low doses of radiation. You may remember, a few years ago, adverse publicity about mammography gave some women the false impression that mammography is a hazard. The misunderstanding arose in Canada when a massive study was launched to compare mammography with physical examination (feeling the breast for lumps) as a means of detecting early breast cancer. The study is designed to determine if it would be worthwhile to screen women with mammography and if doctors should recommend it on a regular basis as they order the now-familiar Pap test for cervical cancer. But when the study began, a few doctors warned, on TV and in newspapers, that women should not subject themselves to repeated mammography because of the danger of radiation.

Unfortunately, some women who heard these warnings became frightened of mammography and are now reluctant to undergo it when their doctors order it as part of an investigation for breast cancer. It is an important diagnosis tool. You have no need to fear that having mammography will harm you. It may save your health.

Having mammography annually is quite safe providing the equipment used is not old and out-dated. All the medical centres taking part in the Canadian study use equipment that gives much lower levels of radiation than were formerly used. Whether mammography will prove effective as a way of screening women for breast cancer and, if so, whether earlier diagnosis will save lives, awaits the outcome of the Canadian study. It involves fourteen medical centres across the country and 90,000 women who have volunteered to take part. Half of them have mammograms each year and half are examined physically. All are taught to examine their own breasts for lumps. It will be a few years before the results are known. The American Cancer Society however, has already recommended annual mammograms for women aged 40 to 59.

Xeroradiography

Xeroradiography, also called a Xeromammography, is a kind of mammogram that combines x-ray with the technology of the Xerox office copier. A special metal plate is exposed to the x-rays and the picture of the breast is printed on paper in blue and white rather than on black and white film. Some medical specialists find a Xeroradiogram shows up a tumour more clearly. However, basically it is the same as mammography.

CAT scan

A scanning device linked to a computer is another machine that lets doctors "see" deep inside the body. Called either a CAT (computerized axial tomography), scanner or CT scanner, it x-rays one thin cross-section of the body after another. It reads, electronically, the information gathered from each fine beam of x-ray as the machine scans the part of the body under examination. All this information is put together in its computer to produce a computerized picture that is displayed on a TV-type screen. It gives a clearer look at soft tissues than conventional x-ray photographs and allows doctors to see tissues behind the ribs or other bones that show as shadows and block the view on regular x-ray pictures.

The machine is large, but a person undergoing a CAT scan feels nothing. The patient simply lies still while the scanner takes many readings. How long a scan takes depends on how much of the body is being examined, but it usually lasts from fifteen minutes to an hour. It might be a total body scan. Each pencil-thin x-ray takes only a few seconds. The scanner will not touch you, but will rotate over you. The total amount of radiation will be no more than from a conventional x-ray and may be less. Usually, you need no special preparation for a CAT scan. It is not a risky procedure and is a great boon to medicine, eliminating the need for much surgery that used to be required for investigation. The CAT scan also allows many patients to avoid painful diagnostic techniques, commonly used in the past.

Ultra-sound

Ultra-sound provides another way of seeing deep into the body without surgery. It is a spin-off of submarine-spotting procedures used during the Second World War, known as sonar. Sound waves, sent through the sea, reflected back signals that indicated when they had struck something solid. From these echo signals, the size of the solid object could be determined, telling sonar operators if it was a submarine. Similarly, an ultra-sound scan, through a device placed against the skin, sends high frequency sound waves into the body, revealing by echoes, what lies beneath. Echoes change as sound waves encounter fluid or air or tissue and the scanner reads these changes. The picture emerges as dots on a screen called an oscilloscope.

No radiation is involved. Indeed ultra-sound is frequently used to monitor the development of an unborn child because it can safely scan the mother's abdomen to show the size and position of the baby.

When it is used to detect a tumour, ultra-sound can show the size and shape of a growth but cannot necessarily distinguish a benign tumour from a cancer tumour. (Research at some centres, such as the Mayo Clinic, Rochester, into computerized ultra-sound, may find ways to make it possible in future to use ultra-sound to distinguish cancer from other growths.) It can tell a solid tumour from a fluid-filled cyst.

An ultra-sound scan causes no pain. It is most frequently used for scans of the abdominal area of the body. The part of the device that touches you is something like a microphone. It is pressed against your skin to send in sound waves that are too high in frequency for you to hear.

Nuclear Magnetic Resonance Imager (NMR)

The newest kind of equipment being used in diagnosis is the NMR (nuclear magnetic resonance imager). The name may confuse lay people because we are accustomed to "nuclear" in the sense of nuclear power. NMR does not involve that. The name comes from the fact that the device makes the nuclei (the central portions) of certain particles in the body, primarily hydrogen particles, resonate, i.e. vibrate and change position. You can't feel it. But by measuring this reaction, the NMR gives doctors information not only about the size, shape and location of tumour tissue, but about the chemistry of cells in the tumour.

The machine consists of a very strong magnet that produces a magnetic field. You are placed on an examining table within this magnetic field. The magnet is so strong that if you carried a credit card into the field, the magnet would erase numbers from it. Yet the amount of energy your body will receive is very small. Studies in several countries over a number of years have shown NMR does not harm body tissue. There is no radiation.

An examination may take anywhere from a few minutes to an hour. The device examines a cross-section, about one centimetre thick, and sends the information to a computer. Each image requires about four minutes. The computer creates the picture. NMR provides a good image of soft tissues. So far NMR is available only at a few large cancer treatment centres, such as Princess Margaret Hospital in Toronto and University of Western Ontario hospitals in London, Ontario. A number of centres in the United States and Britain have also installed NMRs.

Thermography and diaphanography

These two methods, sometimes used in the detection of breast cancer, involve no radiation. However, many doctors do not consider them as reliable as mammography.

Thermography, pioneered in the late 1950s, by a Canadian physician, Dr. Ray Lawson, provides a picture taken with a special camera that shows heat patterns in the breast. A tumour shows up as a hot spot that requires further investigation. Recently, a simplified technique, using a heat-sensitive flexible foil that is laid across the women's chest until colour patterns emerge, has been marketed for use in the offices of general practitioners. However, it has not gained widespread acceptance from doctors.

Diaphanography uses light to display shadows in breasts. The light is held beneath and alongside each breast and the image is displayed on a television monitor screen. When this technique was tested in the late 1970s, it didn't seem particularly useful because it wasn't as accurate as mammography. However, a few doctors believe advances in technology have improved the value of diaphanography. The U.S. National Cancer Institute has said the method may have enough promise to warrant being evaluated scientifically.

Examinations using contrast materials

In some cases, x-rays or scans are used in conjunction with contrast materials that are injected or fed into the body. The materials may be dyes, weak radioactive materials or air. They sharpen the contrast between the organ or tissue being examined and surrounding tissue, producing a clearer picture.

Depending on which organ is under investigation, you may be given the contrast material as a drink or pill to swallow, have it injected by needle, or inserted through a tube. Barium, which is metallic, is one kind of contrast material. A barium enema may be given if the intestines are being examined, for example, or barium might be given in a drink if the upper part of the digestive tract is being investigated. The material coats the inner walls of the tract, so that any growth or tumour on them stands out distinctly.

Dyes may be injected if a moving x-ray is required to enable the doctor to see blood flow or watch an organ in action. Tumours must have blood supplies just like other tissue and sometimes an abnormal pattern of blood vessels will be a tip-off that a tumour is there. In other cases, movie x-rays of blood vessels may be taken to find out if the tumour is obstructing blood flow. Dye in the bloodstream makes flow of blood clearly visible. The movie is called an angiogram. Fluoroscopy is another kind of x-ray movie. It might be used, for example, to observe a lung expanding. Doctors watch the organ in action on a TV-type screen.

If a radioactive material is to be used with a scan, you will probably go to the nuclear medicine department of a hospital to have your testing. Any radioactive material requires skilful handling by specialists in this field. However, you will not be exposed to extensive radiation. The radioactive materials used, called isotopes, give off radiation in such small amounts, a patient gets a dose no larger than from a chest x-ray.

Isotopes show up as dots of light in the image produced by the scanning machine. Tumours are displayed as spots where there are an abnormal number of dots. Such scans are an important way of finding whether there are secondary nests of cells (metastases) in the body.

The most commonly used isotope in the world is technetium-99. A major world supplier of this isotope is Atomic Energy of Canada's Chalk River laboratory in Ontario. It supplies enough of the material to the world each year for twenty million diagnostic tests.

Radioactive iodine is another commonly used isotope, particularly for thyroid, liver and kidney scans.

Endoscopy

Endoscopy is a way of looking into a body passageway with a flexible instrument that can be snaked inside body channels. This technique has replaced many kinds of surgery, once needed for cancer detection and treatment. It was made possible by the development of fibre optics, fine glass fibres that transmit light. With such light attached to a thin instrument that can be inserted into the body, it is possible to see the interior of passageways and some hollow organs, such as the bladder. The doctor looks through an eyepiece, rather as if he or she were looking through a small periscope.

There are a number of these instruments called scopes. Each is named after the part of the body it is designed to examine. For example, a colonoscope is used to examine the colon, a bronchoscope examines the bronchial tubes of the lung, and so forth. Usually, you don't have to be admitted to hospital to have endoscopy. It does not require a general anaesthetic and can be done in an out-patient clinic or doctor's office.

You may be given light sedation to help you relax. There could be a little discomfort. But it will save you from undergoing diagnostic surgery.

As well as looking through a scope to observe the tumour, the doctor may attach a tiny device to the instrument that will brush or snip off samples of cells. These samples will be examined by a pathologist to see if any cells are cancer cells. For example, a small growth called a polyp might be clipped off the wall of the large intestine. Sometimes, though not always, polyps are malignant.

Biopsy

A biopsy is a procedure for taking samples of tissue for examination. There are different ways of getting samples. One is by using a fine needle to draw out a tiny amount of fluid containing clusters of cells. This is called fine needle aspiration. You might compare it with sticking a toothpick into a cake to see if the cake is done, rather than cutting the cake open. It is not always necessary to have the spot where the needle enters "frozen", but in some cases a local anaesthetic is given to numb the site.

Sometimes a wider needle is used, containing a tiny knife that cuts out a pinch of tissue instead of drawing out fluid.

Removing a bit of tissue by surgery is another method. If a whole small tumour is removed it is called excisional biopsy, or in the case of a breast lump, lumpectomy. In some cases, if no cells have spread, an excisional biopsy may cure the cancer. When only part of a tumour can be removed surgically, it is called in incisional biopsy.

The sample obtained will be examined microscopically. Looking at the tissue that has been removed often gives an experienced surgeon a reasonably good idea of whether or not it is cancer, even before it is examined under the microscope. But the final word will come from the pathologist.

Blood and urine tests

No one simple sure test can determine whether a person has cancer in the way that diabetes can be identified from a urine sample. Your doctor will order blood and urine tests largely as part of the assessment of your general state of health.

However, there are some tests that may help in the diagnosis even though they are not foolproof. One blood test, now used world-wide, originated in Canada in the 1960s. Dr. Phil Gold and colleagues at McGill University, Montreal, found a substance in the blood of people with bowel cancer that is not ordinarily found in healthy adults. They called it carcinoembryonic antigen. It is commonly known as CEA. CEA, it turned out, was not specifically connected with bowel cancer.

It is sometimes found in people with other kinds of illnesses. Nevertheless, it provides an indication that further investigation is necessary. Its presence also alerts doctors to a recurrence of cancer in a patient. A rise in CEA levels can indicate a reappearance of the disease long before it can otherwise be detected.

Urine tests may help to detect some kinds of cancer. Blood in urine can be an indication of bladder cancer, although it is also caused by other diseases. Urine is examined with a microscope to detect small red blood cells. It is also tested for protein and sugar, indicators of the patient's state of health.

SYMPTOMS

Different kinds of cancer produce different symptoms. But almost every symptom that might lead a doctor to suspect cancer could be caused by some other ailment. Some people put themselves through unnecessary agony by assuming that they have cancer when they do not. Diagnosing cancer is a complex procedure, calling for extensive and thorough investigation by doctors.

On the following pages, symptoms often associated with particular types of cancer are described. They might lead your doctor to refer you for diagnostic tests. But no one who has any of the symptoms described should think these symptoms automatically indicate the presence of cancer. See your doctor if you have any fears about your health. These sections are intended to help you understand the investigative procedures your doctor may order to search for the cause of the symptoms.

Lung

A persistent, hacking cough in a patient who does not smoke will require further investigation. A doctor will also order tests for a smoker whose cough changes and worsens. Repeated bouts of pneumonia also require looking into, in case it is caused by an airway obstruction. Coughing up blood or a noticeable change in the amount or the appearance of sputum, chest pains or an increased shortage of breath are indications of a need for further examination.

After completing a thorough examination of the patient's general health, the doctor will probably refer a patient with such symptoms to a radiologist to have chest x-rays.

The patient may be asked to collect, each day for three days, sputum samples. Sputum, which is coughed up, contains secretions from the lungs. The patient will be asked to cough into a container and cover the sample with alcohol (gin or vodka will do) to preserve it. The sample will be sent to a laboratory that specializes in the examination of cells. Many lung cancers start in the bronchial tubes (the airways that connect lungs to windpipe) and cells shed by them may be found in sputum.

Bronchoscopy may be required. This involves sliding a thin flexible instrument, a bronchoscope, into each airway, one at a time. Breathing can continue through the second airway, while the examination is in progress. Usually, a local anaesthetic is given to prevent discomfort. If a tumour is seen through the bronchoscope, the surgeon will cut out a sample for microscopic examination.

Pulmonary function tests which measure how well the lungs are working may be part of the investigation. They involve a series of breathing exercises. CAT scans or contrast x-rays may be taken. In some cases, doctors may remove a sample of fluid from the space between the lungs and the chest wall. Usually, a local anaesthetic is used to avoid pain from the needle that is inserted to remove the fluid sample. Sometimes, a small incision is made to allow the insertion of a scope to examine the surface of the lungs and the chest wall or to remove lymph nodes from behind the breast bone. This is done under a general anaesthetic.

Not all the tests described are required by every patient. If lung cancer is detected by means of a sputum test and its location determined by bronchoscopy, the outlook is very favourable. Doctors say at that stage the cancer can frequently be eliminated.

Colon-rectum *(Large intestine)*

The problem with cancer of the large intestine is that it may give no indication it is there for quite a long time. The symptoms may be mistaken for more ordinary digestive complaints or hemorrhoids (piles). Persistent constipation or diarrhoea, chronic gas pains in the lower abdomen, or signs of blood in stool may lead a doctor to investigate the bowel. With a gloved finger, a doctor can examine the final few inches of the rectum which is the lowest section of the colon. He or she feels for polyps, growths that arise from the mucous lining of the intestine. In North America, polyps are extremely common but most of the time are benign. However, because they can become malignant, doctors advise people who produce a lot of polyps to have regular bowel examinations and have the polyps removed.

Hemorrhoids do not become cancerous but they can exist side by side with tumours and, for that reason, it should not be taken for granted that bleeding is caused by hemorrhoids. Bleeding requires investigation.

To examine higher in the intestine than the doctor can reach with a finger, a proctosigmoidoscope or a colonoscope is used. About twelve inches of bowel can be seen through the proctosigmoidoscope. The colonoscope can examine the entire six-foot length of the colon. The invention of the colonoscope brought a vast improvement in the diagnosis of cancer of the colon. It is also used to remove polyps growing on stalks like small toadstools. Polyps that are removed are examined microscopically to make sure they are benign.

Blood in stool is sometimes hidden. It is called "occult" blood. To check for it, a stool sample is examined by means of a Hemoccult test, also called a guaiac test. Most colon cancers bleed. Before the stool is tested, a patient will be asked to follow a meat-free, high bulk (bran and fruits) diet for four days. After the first day, the patient will collect small samples of stool, putting them on a special slide the doctor will provide, which will be sent to a laboratory for examination.

A barium enema may be required. X-rays of the bowel are taken during and after the colon is filled with barium or barium and air to make the picture clearer. It is usual for relaxant drugs to be given to decrease discomfort.

Breast

The majority of breast cancers are found by women themselves. The Cancer Society urges women to learn and practise breast self-examination and an increasing number of women are doing so. At present, however, most women discover breast lumps more or less accidentally.

In 80 per cent of cases, breast lumps are benign. But any lump needs to be investigated. A lump may feel moveable or firmly attached. A moveable lump is likely to be benign.

Other signs that call for investigation are discharge or bleeding from the nipple, puckering or dimpling or pitting of the breast skin, a lump under the arm, an ulcer or sore that won't heal, an inverted nipple if the nipple was previously erect, a change in breast size and, in rare cases, constant breast pain. The most common spot for a suspicious lump is the upper quarter of the breast on the side nearest the arm.

A small number of men develop breast cancer but it is primarily a disease of women. A study published in the British medical journal *The Lancet* in 1981 reported that severe constipation in women may be an indication of the presence of breast disease in certain cases.

Diagnosis will require mammography and probably additional x-rays. A lump will be removed by lumpectomy and analyzed to determine whether it is malignant. Sometimes cells are obtained by needle aspiration biopsy to find out if the lump is a cyst.

In the past, doctors often performed both the biopsy for diagnosis and the mastectomy in one operation. Today women tend to have biopsy only in the process of diagnosis. They await the outcome of laboratory examination of the sample before the decision is made about the extent of surgery required for treatment. The change in breast surgery is described in the chapter on treatment.

Scans, in particular bone and liver scans, and chest x-rays, are done to search for possible spread of breast cancer. Lymph nodes under the arm will be investigated to see if they contain cancer cells. When cancer has been found in the breast, it is imperative to determine whether it has spread beyond the breast because treatment will be quite different if that is the case. If it is confined to one site it can be surgically removed.

A number of cancer surgeons in the United States recommend that women who are considered at high risk of breast cancer have their breasts removed, even if no cancer has been detected in them. This "preventative" surgery is extremely controversial. Women are deemed to be at high risk if their mothers, sisters, or aunts have developed breast cancer at a relatively young age and if their breast tissue is lumpy. The practice has not been widespread in Canada. Doctors who say double mastectomies are warranted as prevention explain that some women are so fearful of breast cancer they become emotionally ill. The surgery not only prevents breast cancer but restores emotional equilibrium. Doctors who believe, on the other hand, that it is unwise to remove healthy tissue, say frequent examinations are a better way to reassure such women and reduce their anxiety.

Cervix

Since the Pap test came into widespread use as a scanning test for cervical cancer, the number of cases of this kind of cancer has been dropping. In British Columbia, for example, where a screening programme began in 1949, there has been a 75 per cent drop in the number of cases. The Pap test involves scraping cells from the cervix, which is the neck of the womb. It is usually done during a routine check-up by a woman's family doctor or gynecologist.

If abnormal cells are found, the physician will notify the patient to come back for a repeat test. Abnormal cells are not necessarily malignant but may appear at risk of becoming cancerous, a condition sometimes called dysplasia.

If there is any indication cancer cells are present, a biopsy will be required. It may be done with an instrument called a colposcope, through which abnormal spots can be looked at and removed.

Symptoms of cervical cancer may include a slight discharge, either watery or bloody, along with irregular menstrual periods, or bleeding or spotting. Low back pain may develop. Constipation, changes in urinating, weight loss or vomiting are other signs to watch for.

If no cancer cells are found by colposcopy but there are symptoms, the patient may be admitted to hospital where a larger sample of tissue will be removed under general anaesthetic. If cancer is found, x-rays, scans or barium enema will likely be ordered to check for spread of cancer.

Uterus

Cancer of the uterus (womb) may be first suspected as the result of a Pap test. However, the test is not nearly as effective in detecting uterine cancer as it is cervical cancer. Cancer of the uterus, also called endometrial cancer because it forms in the lining, the endometrium, typically gives early warning signals. Symptoms may include bleeding between periods or a return of bleeding after menopause. Although there are a number of reasons, other than cancer, that such bleeding may occur, it requires investigation.

An endoscope, a special instrument designed to slip through the cervix into the uterus, is used to collect cells from the lining. Other ways of collecting cells are aspiration curettage, a tube with a syringe to draw out cells, and jet washing, to flush out cell samples. The samples are examined microscopically.

Sometimes diagnosis is made by means of an operation, commonly referred to as a D&C (dilation and curettage) in which the uterus walls are scraped to obtain samples to be analyzed.

Ovary

Cancer of the ovary often gives no indication it is there until a tumour is quite large. It is most often discovered by a physician during a pelvic examination done as part of a routine check-up. The physician may feel the tumour. The majority of ovarian tumours are benign. Both benign and malignant tumours may cause abdominal pain or heaviness, backache or abnormal bleeding. A large tumour can press on the intestines or the urinary tract, causing changes in bowel or bladder habits. Ovarian cysts, which are not cancer, may become as big as tennis balls before they cause any symptoms. Surgery is required to remove the growth and determine its nature. Cancer of the fallopian tubes is rare but not unknown.

Prostate

Sometimes cancer of the prostate has early symptoms, sometimes not. The prostate gland is located just below the bladder and a physician conducting a rectal examination may feel a prostate tumour. Because of the gland's proximity to the tube from the bladder, enlargement of the prostate can interfere with urination. Although enlargement of the prostate is quite common and is not always caused by cancer, medical examination to determine the cause is necessary. Pain in the lower back or thighs may occur if a tumour, either benign or malignant, presses on nerves.

Diagnosis of prostate cancer is made by needle biopsy and x-rays. Often prostate cancer grows slowly and remains localized at the original site. However, a search for possible spread may be needed. Lymph nodes in the groin will probably be examined. Blood tests are also useful because prostate cancer cells may secrete a chemical called acid phosphatase, although not in all cases.

Testes

The earliest indication of a tumour in the testicles is often discomfort or slight enlargement. A dull ache in the scrotum or lower abdomen or groin might be noticed. A mass, either hard or soft, may be felt in the scrotum. Because the testes produce hormones as well as sperm, the breast or nipples may feel tender.

Undescended testicles or those that did not descend until after the age of six have been linked to a greater risk of cancer of the testes. The physician will usually ask the age at which the patient's testicles descended. A tumour may be identified by physical examination, blood tests and urine analysis. A biopsy should *not* be done. Different kinds of scans and x-rays will be required to check for spread because this kind of cancer tends to grow and spread fairly quickly.

Stomach

In the early stages of stomach cancer, symptoms may be so subtle many people, even doctors, consider them ordinary indigestion. A person may think that something he ate didn't agree with him or that he ate too much, making him overly full. When such symptoms continue, investigation is needed. Sometimes the problem is initially believed to be an ulcer. There may be weight loss or unexplained lack of strength. If the tumour has grown large, the doctor may be able to feel it. Endoscopy to view the stomach lining or take samples of cells, washed off the stomach wall by a jet spray of water, helps make the diagnosis. Contrast film, obtained from x-rays taken after the patient has drunk a barium cocktail, may detect the location of the tumour.

Bladder

Blood in the urine may be one of the first indications of bladder cancer, although it is also a symptom of some other kinds of bladder disorders. Urinating may cause a burning sensation and the need to urinate may increase. Pain is not usually an early sign but is likely to develop if the cancer goes undetected. Many bladder tumours turn out to be benign. Urine is analyzed to see if it contains cancer cells. A cystoscope, an instrument designed to slide into the bladder, is used to view the bladder lining and remove samples for laboratory examination. Contrast x-rays, ultra-sound or CAT scans may be required.

Kidney

The combination of back pain, blood in the urine, a lump in the abdomen and weight loss would make a doctor suspect kidney cancer. Kidneys can develop tumours that are not cancer, but tests must be done to find out. Diagnosis may be made by means of a pyelogram, an x-ray taken after dye has been injected into the bloodstream and by x-ray movies of the blood vessels of the kidney. Blood tests, urine analysis and scans may also be needed to determine the nature of the tumour.

In children, cancer of the kidney is most often a kind called Wilms' Tumour, which doctors believe began before birth. It is often discovered by a parent who finds a mass in the child's abdomen, usually on one side only. Painful urination or blood in the urine may also be symptoms. Early diagnosis is crucial, because if the cancer is detected in infancy and treated, the child has every likelihood of growing up healthy.

Pancreas

One of the most difficult cancers to diagnose, because symptoms mimic those of other ailments, cancer of the pancreas may be mistaken for gall-bladder disease. However, advances in scanning techniques have greatly improved diagnosis. The patient may be yellowed from jaundice and have light, clay-coloured stool and dark urine. Other symptoms are weight loss and abdominal pain, often radiating to the back, that is eased by bending forward. Weakness, indigestion or constipation may occur. Methods of diagnosis include CAT scan, ultra-sound and sometimes, a pancreatic function test which involves collecting samples from the intestine after the patient has been put on a special diet or given injections to increase pancreatic secretions. Benign tumours of the pancreas are not uncommon and may produce symptoms similar to malignant tumours. If it is not possible to remove the tumour by surgery, yet it is uncertain whether it is benign or cancerous, a needle biopsy to obtain cells for microscopic study may be required.

Liver

Usually early symptoms of liver cancer are vague and similar to stomach upsets. They include nausea, vomiting, a feeling of pressure in the abdomen, and constipation. Jaundice, weight loss, fever, or a pain that radiates to the right shoulder blade may occur. The liver may feel hard and tender and be enlarged. Such symptoms in a person with chronic liver disease, such as hepatitis or cirrhosis, would make a doctor particularly suspicious of liver cancer. Blood tests may reveal changes in levels of calcium in the blood. Investigation will probably include scans, x-ray movies of blood vessels in the organ and biopsy. Cancer of the liver, while common in some parts of Africa and Asia, is relatively rare in North America. In most cases, when cancer is found in the liver in a Canadian or American patient, it is a secondary cancer that has spread there from another site.

Gall-bladder

Symptoms of this rare cancer might suggest gall-stones. Certain foods can cause indigestion. Jaundice, vomiting, loss of appetite and weakness are possible signs. Diagnosis is made by CAT scan or ultra-sound.

Leukemias

There are different kinds of leukemia but all involve abnormal production of white cells in the blood. In children and young adults, the most common kind is acute lymphocytic leukemia, commonly referred to as ALL. It usually appears suddenly, seeming like a cold with fatigue and malaise that steadily grow worse. Because ALL interferes with blood clotting, prolonged bleeding from a minor wound or easy bruising can occur. Pinpoint spots of blood, called petechiae, may show up on the skin looking rather like a rash. Sometimes a dentist is the first to notice unusual bleeding of the gums. A sore throat, night sweats, weight loss, susceptibility to infection and pain in the joints may also be symptoms.

In adults, chronic lymphocytic leukemia and acute myelogenous leukemia are the most common kinds. Chronic myelogenous leukemia is rarer. Chronic leukemias usually show up more gradually than acute leukemias. However, the symptoms may be similar. In adults, leukemia may be detected first by a routine blood test.

Diagnosis of leukemia is made by blood count tests, performed in laboratories with computerized equipment capable of determining rapidly the number of each kind of white blood cells in the blood. The disease causes an abnormal number of immature white cells. Because blood cells originate in bone marrow, a sample of bone marrow is taken by needle biopsy, usually done on the hipbone.

Lymphomas

Hodgkin's disease is one kind of lymphoma. But the group of cancers called non-Hodgkin's lymphomas are more common. Hodgkin's disease may first show up as a swollen lymph gland, typically in the neck, that remains swollen. Swollen glands caused by infections are very common but the enlargement rarely lasts three weeks or more. A gland that stays swollen for that long requires investigation. In some, but not the majority of patients, lymph nodes become painful after drinking alcohol. Hodgkin's disease is distinguished from other lymphomas by the presence of an abnormal type of cell called Reed-Sternberg cells. Other symptoms of lymphomas are: backache, swelling of the legs, fever, night sweats, nausea, relentless fatigue and itching.

Diagnosis requires extensive testing. Accurate determination of the stage (degree of severity) of lymphoma is critical in order to plan the treatment. Investigation may include physical examination of lymph nodes, blood and urine tests, bone marrow tests, a variety of x-rays, lymphography which involves injecting dye into the lymph system so it can be observed by x-ray, biopsy of a node and scans. Not all these kinds of diagnostic procedures will be required for any one patient, but diagnosis will require a combination of tests.

Multiple Myeloma

The first sign of this cancer of blood plasma cells is usually deep-seated pain in bones, especially the back. The pain may come and go but gets worse with exercise. Swelling of the ribs, weight loss, bones that break without apparent reasons may also be signs. Multiple Myeloma is commonly known to Europeans as Kahler's Disease and it is also called plasma cell myeloma. The cancer cells destroy bone. Diagnosis involves blood and urine tests to check for abnormal proteins. X-rays of bone may disclose bone loss in spots. The disease begins in the bone marrow and usually a needle biopsy of marrow is taken to confirm the diagnosis.

Brain

Both benign and malignant brain tumours cause a wide variety of symptoms, including headache, muscle weakness on one side of the body, failing or double vision, lack of balance or personality changes. Convulsions or seizures might occur. Cancer of the brain is not common. However, benign tumours are also often dangerous because the tight fit of the skull gives a tumour no room in which to grow and it may press on brain tissue.

Diagnosis is usually made by CAT scan, sometimes after an iodine-like dye has been injected into the bloodstream so that blood vessels in the tumour will show up more clearly. Movie x-rays of blood vessels are sometimes taken. Vision and hearing tests may be part of the examination.

Central nervous system

In children, the second most common cancer, after leukemia, is neuroblastoma which often begins in nerve cells of the adrenal gland. Usually, before the age of four, the child develops a firm, irregular-shaped mass in the abdomen. It is often first noticed by a parent bathing the child. Lymph nodes may be enlarged, the child may lose weight, be pale or run a temperature. Examination of the child and blood and urine tests help make the diagnosis.

Pharynx *(Throat)*

Early cancer of the pharynx sometimes causes no obvious symptoms. The first indication may be enlargement of lymph nodes. Sometimes nosebleeds, difficulty in swallowing or breathing or pain in the throat cause the patient to seek medical attention. Diagnosis is made by biopsy of the tumour. Cancer of the tonsils at first can seem like an ordinary sore throat. Pain may radiate to one ear. A lump in the neck is an indication it is not a run-of-the-mill sore throat.

Larynx *(Vocal Cords)*

Hoarseness is the most common early sign and becomes increasingly worse. The patient may feel a constant need to clear the throat of sticky mucus. Usually there is no cough. Difficulty in breathing or swallowing may occur. Nodules that are not cancer can develop on the vocal cords of people who overuse their voices. These are sometimes called Screamer's nodules. However, a biopsy may be needed to rule out cancer. Abnormal spots, other than nodules, are examined by laryngoscopy, which involves sliding a thin flexible instrument down the throat to look at the larynx.

Esophagus *(Food tube)*

Early symptoms include difficulty in swallowing solid foods and a feeling of pressure beneath the breast bone. Thirst, cough, excessive production of saliva in the mouth, weight loss and sometimes chest pain, are other symptoms. Diagnosis is made by x-ray and endoscopy. A brush attached to the instrument used to look into the esophagus, sweeps up cells to be examined microscopically, or a bit of tissue may be snipped off for analysis.

Mouth, tongue and lip

Whitish, thickened spots on the mouth are often noticed first. They may not be cancer but they should be investigated. In some cases, patches in the mouth are dark in colour. Sores on lip or tongue that don't heal should be seen by a doctor. Unexplained bleeding in the mouth or numbness and stiffness of the jaw muscle that makes chewing difficult are signs.

To investigate abnormal spots in the mouth, the doctor scrapes cells from them for analysis. If the smear of cells suggests malignancy, the spot is biopsied for further study.

Lip tumours, most often found on the lower lip, are often benign but need to be examined to rule out cancer. Cancer of the tongue, frequently along the edge and looking like small sores or ulcers, may be slightly painful. Cancer at the back of the tongue may cause a sore throat with pain spreading to the ears.

Because lip and tongue cancers are visible in most cases, they are detected early.

Skin

The most common of all cancers, skin cancer, may show itself in various ways: as a change in the colour or size of a pigmented spot; as a pearly nodule that keeps getting bigger; as a raised red or dark patch; or as changes in a mole.

The two most frequent, and readily curable, kinds are called basal cell carcinoma and squamous cell carcinoma. Removing them is both the way of obtaining a sample for diagnosis and a cure.

Malignant melanoma is cancer of the pigment cells. It is usually considered a skin cancer, although it can occur in pigment in the eye as well as in the skin. It is relatively rare, although the number of cases in the United States is increasing. It may show up as a new mole or as a change in a mole already there. A mole that suddenly begins growing, bleeding, becomes inflamed, or has a bluish cast or a halo of pigment around it, should be seen immediately by a doctor.

Occasionally a wart or a basal cell carcinoma may be mistaken for malignant melanoma.

When possible, the mole is totally removed. If all of it cannot be removed, a part of it is taken for microscopic examination. Blood tests, blood counts, x-rays and scans may be required to track down any possible spread.

STAGING OF CANCER

As well as making the diagnosis of cancer from tests and examinations, doctors determine the extent of the disease. You may have been puzzled to hear a cancer described as Stage I or Stage IV ori by letters and numbers such as T1, NO, MO. It is medical shorthand that defines the size of the tumour and whether it has spread to lymph nodes or elsewhere. The letter T stands for Tumour, N for nodes and M for metastasis.

Most kinds of cancer are divided into four stages: Stage I indicates no spread has been found. There are variations in the classifications of different cancers but in general the higher the number, the more extensive the disease. For example, in breast cancer T1 means the tumour is less than two centimetres in size. NO indicates no spread to the lymph nodes and MO means no spread to distant sites.

Staging is extremely important in determining the kind of treatment required.

Fourteen
Treatment

WEIGHING OPTIONS

The kinds of treatment used today all have one goal—to get cancer cells out of the body.

Someday, in the future, there may be ways to turn cancer cells back into normal cells. Doctors can do that in the laboratory. Dr. Leo Sachs of Israel first demonstrated it was possible to reverse the cancer process in leukemia cells growing in cultures. But it is not yet known how to do the same thing in a patient's body.

There are three major ways of getting rid of cancer cells: by surgery; by destroying the cells with radiation; or by killing them with drugs (chemotherapy). Often treatment involves a combination of two of the three or all three.

The method used depends on the kind of cancer and how far it has advanced when it is detected. In some instances, it may also depend on which treatment a patient chooses. If decisions are to be made, a patient should know what types of treatment are possible.

But some people have out-of-date or distorted ideas about the three main methods of therapy. To see them in historical perspective may help you discover how much they have advanced.

Surgery is the oldest of the treatments. From ancient times, doctors cut out tumours they could see on skin or other body surfaces. But it was late in the 19th century before surgery was attempted to remove unseen tumours.

The first cancer surgery developed was the radical mastectomy for breast cancer. It was a drastic operation that often left women with disabled arms and disfigured torsos. But for the first time, breast cancer in some women was cured.

At the time, doctors did not know why it worked for some women while others continued to have cancer in their bodies. They didn't understand how cancer spreads. But it was the start of surgical removal of many kinds of tumours.

Radiation therapy began in the 1920s after it became known that x-rays could destroy cells. The early x-ray treatment machines had low power that made treatment difficult and unpleasant. They often caused skin burns. These machines could not shoot x-rays deep into the body. It was not until the 1950s that dramatic improvement in radiation therapy would come about.

Drugs or chemicals to combat cancer came, in large measure, out of the Second World War. Dr. Charles Huggins of Chicago found that the female hormone, estrogen, could shrink prostate tumours in men (a discovery that won him a Nobel prize) just before the war but the cancer drugs of today were unimagined until, in 1943, a ship carrying mustard gases was blown up in Naples harbour and many people exposed to the gases died. The gases, it was found, had destroyed cells of lymph glands and bone marrow, raising the question: Could mustard gases be harnessed to kill cancer cells? They could. Nitrogen mustard is still a common cancer drug today.

By mid-century, effective treatments were beginning to emerge but, for the most part, physicians treating cancer patients found it distressing and disheartening. With antibiotics in their black bags, doctors could be miracle workers among patients with bacterial infections once considered fatal, but cancer remained a formidable foe. Recalling the 1950s, one doctor said candidly: "We were probably doing a worse job in helping cancer patients than physicians early in the century had done. They dealt with a lot of diseases they couldn't cure and cancer was just one of them. They provided compassionate care because it was all they had to offer. We could cure diseases like tuberculosis and pneumonia that used to kill people. But we were no longer comfortable dealing with diseases we couldn't cure. Cancer made us feel like failures. I think we often left our patients feeling that we'd abandoned them."

Some of us may remember older relatives being treated for cancer when doctors had little to offer patients. Much has changed since then—treatments, doctors' attitudes and even patients' expectations are different today. Consumers today, including consumers of medical care, expect to be informed. Many patients want to take part in deciding which treatment they should undergo, if there are options, and seek full explanations of the risks and benefits.

Not every patient wants to be involved in making such decisions, however, and if someone we love has cancer we must remember it is the patient's right to put his or her care entirely in the hands of the doctors. When cancer is diagnosed, it may feel as if the plane one is flying has plummetted and the patient desperately wants an experienced pilot to grab the controls. You or I might want to make our own choices about treatment, but some patients need their doctors to make all decisions and to tell them only as much as necessary.

If you are faced with treatment choices, you may find weighing the alternatives far from easy. Doctors themselves often have different opinions about what is best.

For example, there is no consensus in the medical profession on the best treatment for early breast cancer. The radical mastectomy, devised in 1894 by Dr. William Halsted of Baltimore, Maryland, remained the accepted treatment for forty years. It removed the breast, the muscle underneath the breast, and lymph glands and usually required skin grafts. But as better understanding of cancer developed, some doctors began switching to less mutilating surgery. In 1939 in Toronto, Dr. Vera Peters, a radiologist who pioneered in breast-saving treatment, began keeping records to compare conservative surgery that removed only the tumour plus radiation treatment with mastectomy. Thirty years later, she was able to publish results that showed long-term survival rates were virtually the same for both treatments.

Elsewhere in North America, doctors were gradually accepting simple mastectomy, removing only the breast, as treatment for early cases. It did not cure any more women than Halsted's radical operation, but it spared many women the grief of disability and deformity. Today, fewer than three per cent of patients in North America undergo radical mastectomies.

At the same time, particularly in Canada where doctors took the lead in adopting partial mastectomy or lumpectomy, even simple mastectomies began to be replaced by lumpectomies. One Toronto doctor calls a lumpectomy "the women's lib operation" because women seeking mastery over their own bodies began to insist on it rather than lose a breast. It leaves the breast looking quite normal apart from a small scar.

But not all surgeons believe lumpectomy is safe. Tumours may crop up in the part of the breast that remains. When breasts that have been removed are examined for microscopic tumours, pathologists have sometimes found tiny tumours in them, too small to be seen on x-ray or felt. Some doctors, therefore, are unwilling to leave breast tissue in case tiny tumours are lurking in it, and they encourage patients to have mastectomies.

A woman needs to consider whether she is willing to take the risk when she is choosing between mastectomy and lumpectomy.

Some women who have lumpectomies also undergo radiation therapy in case any cancer calls remain. Others do not.

A study at two Toronto hospitals examined the outcomes of treatment for more than 1,000 women treated since 1958 of whom some had no radiation after lumpectomy, some had radiation to the one breast and some had radiation to both breasts and lymph nodes. No difference was found in survival rates among the three groups and no difference in the number of women who developed tumours in lymph nodes later. But it did find that tumours arose in the remaining part of the breast that had been operated on, in twice as many women who had no radiation therapy.

One might think that is sufficient evidence that lumpectomy followed by radiation is preferable. But the study did not end there. Women who developed second tumours had second lumpectomies and in the long run, they did as well and had no greater risk of dying than the women who received radiation.

Further studies are now underway involving hospitals

throughout the province of Ontario because it is not yet clear which treatment is better. It is possible that some women should have radiation and others may not need it. The study may make this clear and if it does doctors will know which patients need radiation. Until that occurs, the choice is difficult, even for women with full information. When one Toronto doctor asked eight women, four doctors and four nurses, which way they would select for themselves, four came down on each side, with two doctors and two nurses on each, evenly split on whether they would choose radiation after lumpectomy.

Weighing options can be equally difficult for patients with other kinds of cancer. Patients with bone cancer may have to decide between losing a leg to surgery or to have less surgery, take drugs and undergo radiation. Those with rectal cancer may need to choose between surgery and radiation therapy.

Many of us are unaccustomed to making decisions about matters so complex. Patients need time to absorb much new information when treatment strategy is being planned. Cancer forces a patient to be sharply aware that life is a tightrope on which one is not allowed to stand still, immobile. While it is important that treatment get underway reasonably quickly, no patient should feel so rushed or pressured by family or physician, that he or she cannot think clearly.

"I took a long time to get over my resentment and anger that my breast was removed," one woman said several years after her mastectomy. "I'm sure if it had been my own decision I'd have felt differently. Yes, I agreed to it although I had heard about lumpectomies. But everything happened too fast for me to get myself sorted out about what I wanted."

A patient may have heard horror stories about treatments that would frighten the wits out of anybody. There are people and organizations who bitterly oppose conventional medical therapy and actively spread the word that cancer surgery is butchery, radiation is burning and chemotherapy is poisoning. Their motives vary. Their beliefs may be genuine or self-serving, but they may convince some patients to reject treatment.

No reputable doctor would claim the treatments we have today are perfect. A relentless search goes on for better ones. It is true cancer treatments are not like therapies given for minor ailments, but cancer is not a minor ailment. When it is hit hard by treatment, some of the blows may land on a patient's body in unwanted ways. Nevertheless, a person who is more frightened of treatment than of the disease has possibly heard only of the downside and not talked to patients who have come through courses of treatment free of cancer.

The following sections may help you understand the various kinds of treatment and what to expect if you are scheduled to undergo them.

Surgery

Like all kinds of operations, cancer surgery is safer today because of improved anaesthetics and well-trained anaesthetists. It is also much more precise, thanks to the enormous improvements in diagnostic equipment. Whereas surgeons in the past could seldom be sure of the nature of a tumour before they operated, today with scans and fibre optic instruments to examine the tumour beforehand, they have a much more accurate picture.

Surgery is usually considered the best approach when a tumour can be removed completely. It may be the only treatment needed if cells from the tumour have not spread to other parts of the body. Depending on where a tumour is located, surgeons may be able to remove the growth or the organ that contains it.

Nature has given us a surplus of some tissues, including organs that come in pairs. A person can live normally with one lung or one kidney if the other must be removed. We can manage without a stomach or a uterus or a gall-bladder. Other organs have the capacity to regenerate rapidly to replace what is removed.

If it were not for cancer's rotten trick of shipping out cells to other parts of the body, surgery alone could cure many cancers. "Cancer is like blowing a dandelion, scattering seedlings," explains one cancer nurse. "You may not see where the seeds land but you know each one can grow a new plant." Surgery is like digging up the dandelion plant. You get rid of it but it may have scattered seeds before you dug it. If there is reason to suspect that has happened, radiation or chemotherapy or both may be needed following the operation.

In recent years, treatment has tended to involve more conservative surgery with surgeons removing less tissue while radiation or chemotherapy has been added in case there are cancer cells that have moved away from the primary tumour. For example, surgeons are sometimes able to save the legs of patients with sarcomas in bone or connective tissue. They remove only the tumour instead of amputating the leg and the patients receive drug and radiation therapy. Studies at the U.S. National Cancer Institute and in centres in California and Alabama found nine in ten such patients could be left with useful legs and the risk of cancer reappearing in the saved leg was small.

However, it is not yet known whether these patients will continue to remain free of cancer in the long run. More years must go by before we find out. The extent of the risk of saving a patient's leg is not yet known. A patient making the decision in partnership with his doctor today faces a tough choice with few facts on which to base it.

Less extensive surgery is also possible for a number of cancers, because of the invention of flexible fibreoptics instruments such as the colonoscope and bronchoscope. To these, tiny surgical knives can be attached that are unsheathed after the instrument is inserted in the body passageway. The doctor can see small tumours through the eyepiece of the scope and remove them with the little knife. Such surgery is most commonly used in the removal of polyps from the large intestine. They are not always malignant but doctors believe they should be removed anyway because colon cancer often starts in them. "A fight against polyps is a fight against cancer," says one medical specialist.

In the past, surgery (colostomy) was the acceptable treatment for cancers of the rectum and anal canal. Most patients who underwent surgery had to have an artificial opening created, through which body waste emptied into a small pouch or bag. Now radiation, sometimes combined with chemotherapy, is gradually replacing surgery so patients are not left with the inconvenience of a stoma (the new opening).

A report on changes in surgery by the American College of Surgeons says: "In the 1980s few patients with anal canal cancers will require radical surgery and permanent colostomy." In Toronto, some patients with rectal cancer who refused surgery have been treated by radiation. The rectum, of which the anal canal is the final segment, presents a steady target for the radiation beam. However, above that the colon is in constant motion and radiation cannot be be used. Doctors are beginning to believe it is worthwhile to try radiation first on rectal cancer because, should it fail to be effective, they have surgery in reserve. The operation can still be done.

When a permanent colostomy is unavoidable, today there are pouches of superior design that makes them invisible. "You could wear a bikini if you wanted," says one member of the United Ostomy Association, an organization of patients with stomas who help new patients adapt. (See directory of organizations at the end of the book).

One field of surgery in which remarkable advances have been made is reconstructive surgery. Patients who have had tumours removed, particularly from the face, can now have cheeks or jaws restored with living tissue from their own bodies. Micro-surgery has made it possible. Working with the aid of surgical microscopes, surgeons who specialize in the field stitch blood vessels and nerves as fine as hairs. It enables them to move living muscle, tissue and skin from the torso to the face to create near-normal features. One woman who had part of her jaw and most of her cheek removed says, "I thought I would spend the rest of my life as a recluse not wanting anybody to see me. I wondered if life would be worth living." She was astonished at how like herself she looked after facial reconstruction and within a short time she felt so comfortable in public she returned to her part-time job at a neighbourhood store.

For other patients, missing features may be replaced with artificial ones that are sculpted and matched in colour by medical artists so skilful they make disfigurement vanish.

Breast replacement is becoming common as more women request it and as surgeons become less insistent on removing skin covering breast tissue. The most usual of several techniques is the implanting of silicone under the skin. A new nipple may be fashioned by using a segment of the other one.

Another method is to shift tissue from elsewhere on the woman's body to replace the missing breast. If a patient wants this done, she should discuss it in advance with her surgeon. Usually the surgeon will call in a plastic surgeon to plan the operation. The plastic surgeon will do the breast reconstruction after the mastectomy. Sometimes reconstruction is done immediately following breast removal, sometimes later after healing of the mastectomy wound.

One kind of breast reconstruction, still considered experimental, involves moving skin, tissue and muscle with its blood supply from the woman's abdomen to fashion a new breast immediately after mastectomy. One plastic surgeon who performs this operation says: "The patient knows she is rid of cancer, that she has a new breast and a flatter belly as a bonus all at the same time and psychologically that's a big plus."

Some doctors, however, fear that immediate breast reconstruction might hide a recurrence of cancer or that cancer could develop in skin that is left to cover an implant. They believe an artificial, removable breast (prosthesis) is a safer replacement. The Cancer Society in your area may have a list of suppliers in the community from whom you can obtain a prosthesis. There are several different kinds.

It must be the woman's decision whether to have breast reconstruction, although if she is having chemotherapy, she may be required to wait until the course of treatment has ended.

For women who would be devastated emotionally by the loss of a breast, the benefit of restoration may far outweigh the risk. Male doctors used to consider a woman excessively vain if she found losing a breast unbearable, but the majority of surgeons have come to realize the patient's distress is not simply vanity. She may fear losses of sexuality, femininity and love that will shatter her life.

As well as the familiar surgery to remove tumours, you may hear of chemosurgery, cryosurgery and laser surgery.

Chemosurgery involves painting a paste-like chemical on a

tumour to destroy the outer layer of cells and repeating this treatment, layer after layer, until the tumour is gone. It is primarily a treatment for tumours in places like the eyelid where it would be difficult to cut away a tumour by conventional surgery.

Cryosurgery is a freezing technique. It turns tumour cells into ice with liquid nitrogen. Sometimes used on skin tumours, it is also being tested experimentally on cancers of the pancreas, head and bone.

Laser surgery is the elimination of cells with light beams that are like knives of pin-point precision. The uses of laser surgery are increasing steadily. Among other things, it is being used to erase tumours that are blocking tubes and ducts in the body. People with cancer of the esophagus, whose general health is too poor to allow them to undergo the rigours of radiation, have had laser surgery to clear tumours that are interfering with swallowing.

Many people in the world have been successfully treated with surgery for cancers of the large intestine, breast, cervix, thyroid, uterus, bladder, kidney and skin. But surgery cannot work against cancers that are not solid tumours or when tumours are embedded in tissue the body can't do without. Then doctors turn to other weapons to try to conquer cancer.

Radiation

Some people think, wrongly, that if radiation is required it must mean their cancer is advanced and life-threatening, that this is a last resort. Far from it. In fact, more than half of all cancer patients are treated with radiation, either by itself or in combination with surgery and drugs, and many of them are restored to health.

Most of us know less about radiation therapy than we do about surgery. There is little reason to become acquainted with it unless one encounters cancer. Unlike surgery, radiation is not used as treatment for many kinds of diseases. Nurses and doctors at treatment centres are aware of this and know patients will have many questions. You will probably find they make every effort to provide opportunities for you to ask about everything you don't understand. The staff members realize the machines they use look huge and intimidating to people who haven't seen them before and that patients are naturally apprehensive about how they work. It is normal to feel anxious when you face the unknown. But stress is lessened when you know what to expect. No patient or relative should hesitate to ask for information.

Radiation therapy has improved tremendously over the past thirty years. Both equipment and the techniques used have come a long way since the 1930s, when radiation was in its infancy. X-ray machines used were still low powered twenty years later.

Among the first scientists in the world to recognize the possibility of developing high energy radioactive sources was Canada's Dr. Harold Johns. Low power machines could not put x-rays deep into the body without causing burns. Dr. Johns's work with x-rays began during the Second World War and continued afterwards at the University of Saskatchewan. From his research came treatment with radioactive cobalt, usually called cobalt 60. The first cobalt machine built was used in a Saskatoon hospital. It was the prototype model on which cobalt machines were patterned. The world's first commercial cobalt 60 unit was built by Atomic Energy of Canada and was installed in Victoria Hospital, London, Ontario in 1951.

This was the start of a new era in radiation therapy. Radiation could now penetrate the body to reach deep tumours. The word "cobalt" became virtually a synonym for radiation. Even today, patients often say they are getting cobalt treatment although the machines used to treat them actually contain no cobalt. There are other radiation machines today, more powerful than cobalt 60 units, but the cobalt units, solid and reliable, are still in use too. Cobalt machines emit gamma rays, which have the same properties as x-rays, while the newer linear accelerators produce x-rays.

Linear accelerators were developed in the 1960s. They contain no radioactive material like cobalt, but instead produce x-rays by speeding electrons down a long tube to strike a plate which causes the creation of x-rays. The first generation of linear accelerators was not much more powerful than cobalt machines. But over the next twenty years, new technology, such as transistors and microchips, made it possible to manufacture accelerators that put out much more energy.

Toronto's Princess Margaret Hospital was one of the first places in the world to treat patients with a second generation accelerator capable of beaming larger doses of radiation into tumours with minimal damage to tissues it passed through en route. Again, the skill of Dr. Johns made it possible. He modified an industrial accelerator that had not been designed for cancer treatment so that it could be used to help cancer patients.

Since then these new-style machines have come on the market. One of the best, Atomic Energy of Canada's Therac 25, is used in a number of centres in Canada and the United States. The first Therac 25s were installed in Toronto's Sunnybrook Medical Centre cancer clinic and in Nova Scotia's Cancer Treatment and Research Foundation clinic in Halifax in 1984.

Whether a patient is treated on a cobalt 60 machine or a linear accelerator may depend on the kind of cancer. But other factors, such as the individual's build, are taken into consideration. Two patients with similar cancers may be treated on different machines. It does not mean one patient's disease is more serious than the other's.

There is another kind of accelerator called a cyclotron, but only a relatively few patients are likely to undergo its treatment in the near future. One cyclotron, called TRIUMF, is being tested at the University of British Columbia, Vancouver, and others are located in a few centres such as Lawrence Berkeley Laboratory in California and Harvard University, Cambridge, Massachusetts in the United States. A cyclotron makes a different kind of radiation by creating sub-atomic particles. The particles produced by the Vancouver machine are called pions or pimesons.

It is hoped pions will prove useful against brain tumours that are out of reach of conventional radiation because they are hidden behind dense protective skull bone. But use of cyclotrons is still under investigation and their value will not be known until a few years down the line.

Basically, what radiation therapy does is hit tumour cells with high energy rays to break the cells' genetic material, chromosomes. The genetic material is like a two-stranded coiled ribbon and x-rays cut the ribbon like scissors. Breaking the genetic material can prevent a cell from reproducing itself. (Pi-mesons hit the genetic material with what has been called a depth-charge effect, rather than cutting it like x-rays, but the purpose is the same.)

Normal cells in the line of fire may also be hit. But cells are most vulnerable to x-ray damage when they are dividing into two cells and genetic material is uncoiled and copying itself. Most of the time normal cells are not dividing, while cancer cells are. Cancer is constant production of more cells. Furthermore, normal cells have better repair mechanisms with which to mend themselves if they are hit and they can survive while cancer cells die.

Great advances have also been made in planning treatment strategy so radiation bull's-eyes a precise target. "Now we can put the dose required into almost any site in the body," explains one top radiation specialist.

Radiation emitted by machines, called external beam radiation, is by far the more common method but it is possible to give radiation therapy through implants. It is called internal radiation therapy. Small amounts of radioactive material are placed in the patient's body, either in a cavity or directly into the tumour where it is left for a few days. When this method is used, the patient is required to stay in hospital, whereas people receiving external beam radiation don't usually need to be hospitalized.

If you are to have radiation treatment (external beam), this is what you can expect. Treatment won't start on your first visit to the treatment centre because it must be carefully planned. You will meet the doctor in charge of your therapy and other members of the team. The doctor is a radiation therapist or radiation oncologist. Radiation therapy is also called radiotherapy, x-ray therapy, irradiation or cobalt. Don't let it confuse you, they all mean the same.

You will have a number of tests to help the doctor assess your disease and determine the best treatment strategy. It may take three or four visits before planning is completed. On the team are a clinical physicist who has special expertise in machine use, a dosimetrist, who calculates the dose of radiation, radiographers, who help in planning, a radiation technologist who will run the machine and give the treatment and a specially trained nurse.

You may not meet all team members. Some work behind the scenes. But you will become well acquainted with your technologist and nurse and find them excellent sources of information. They will be with you to explain your treatment as you go along.

Radiation is measured in units called "centiGrays," or "rads" which stands for radiation absorbed dose and is the amount of radiation taken in by the tissue. The dose you receive will depend on a number of factors, such as the type of cancer, where it is located, your size and your general health.

Using special ink, your doctor will mark lines on your skin identifying the exact area to be treated. You'll be told not to wash them off. They are important for targeting the treatment. Should they come off accidentally, do *not* try to redraw them yourself. The slightest error could be harmful to you.

As part of the planning, a machine called a simulator may be used. It looks like a treatment machine but it is not. It's a special x-ray machine that simulates energy beams hitting the target, to provide therapists with a way to ensure their planned doses will be right on the mark before actual treatment begins. Some patients, particularly those with head or neck tumours, may have masks or helmets molded to fit that they will wear during each treatment. They prevent any slight alteration of the patient's position during treatment. Not all patients need them. It depends where the tumour is.

Patients who are to receive radiation to the head or neck or whole body will need to see a dentist who will teach them mouth care. Radiation can weaken the structure of teeth and patients may need to apply fluoride daily for the rest of their lives.

When planning is complete, you'll be told which machine will be used and how many treatments are scheduled. There is no set number of treatments. It varies from patient to patient, even among those with similar cancers. Some patients may be able to take a larger dose each time and require a fewer number of sessions. It does not mean your cancer is more serious if you are prescribed a greater number of treatments than another patient with your kind of cancer. The number of treatments is not an indication of the severity of disease.

Usually, patients receive treatment five days a week for a number of weeks. Four or five weeks is about average. Treatment takes only a couple of minutes. You feel nothing. The first time you may wonder if you've been treated at all. "I thought I'd feel a burning or heating sensation or something," said one man. "I thought maybe the machine wasn't working when I didn't feel anything from it." Most patients quickly get accustomed to the large size of the machine and the whirring noise it makes.

You may feel somewhat scared to learn you will be left alone in the room while you get your treatment. The radiotherapy technician giving the treatment will be able to see you through a window or on a TV screen and will talk to you by means of an intercom. The technician cannot stay beside you because, in the course of a day's work, he or she would receive excessive and dangerous doses of radiation. You may notice they wear badges that measure how much radiation they have been exposed to. The badges are safeguards to warn of levels that could be harmful.

If you smoke you may be asked to forego cigarettes for six to eight hours before treatment. Studies show smoking may reduce the benefits of radiation.

You will be asked to lie still during the two to four minutes of treatment. The machine is positioned so its beam is directed at the tumour. It can be moved up and down or around so radiation can hit the tumour from different angles. You will be advised to try and relax and to breathe normally.

Generally patients can go home or back to work after each treatment. If your home town is too far from the centre to allow daily commuting, inquire about special accommodation for patients. Patient lodges have been established near a number of treatment centres. They provide nursing care, should you need it, as well as meals and companionship. Often helpful programmes are offered, such as meetings you can attend to learn about nutrition or patient groups in which to share feelings. In Canada, the cost of staying in such a lodge is not covered by Medicare but it may be paid fully or in part for you by a provincial cancer foundation or provincial cancer society. Your local Cancer Society branch is a good source of information.

So much publicity has been given to the hazards of radioactive waste and to public uproars over where to dump such materials, it is hardly surprising that many people, including patients, worry about radioactive emissions from the bodies of people who have radiation therapy. Those worries are groundless. You have no cause to think you will be any danger to others during your treatment.

Some patients have asked if they should use paper plates at home rather than family dishes to avoid contaminating others, or if their clothing becomes radioactive or if they should keep their distance from family members. The answers are no, no and no! You need to do nothing different at all. You are not a walking radiation source.

The situation is different, however, for patients who have internal radiation therapy. The radioactive material, put into their bodies in capsules, seeds or needles, does give off radiation. While the implant is in place, the patients stay in hospital and usually limits are put on how long visitors may spend with them. Pregnant women may be advised not to visit. Nurses take special precautions to protect themselves while they are providing care to these patients. Once the implant is removed, however, the patient is no hazard to others. The radioactivity is gone. It was the implant that was the only hazard, not the patient's body.

Among cancers that may be treated with implants are cervix, tongue, and in some centres, breast, following partial mastectomy. The radioactive materials may be cobalt, radium, cesium gold or phosphorous.

External beam radiation has made dramatic inroads against

Hodgkin's disease. It is used alone in early cases and in combination with chemotherapy in more advanced cases. In the past ten years, the percentage of patients successfully treated for early Hodgkin's disease has risen from 68 per cent to 90 per cent and in patients with more advanced disease, from 10 per cent to 70 per cent.

Radiation therapy has also proved highly effective, in combination with chemotherapy, against cancer of the testes. Few men with testicular cancer die of their disease today.

Both Hodgkin's disease and testicular cancer tend to occur in young people, so the big improvement in treatment is particular cause for jubilation.

Prostate cancer, at one time, was almost always treated surgically. But now early prostate cancer is likely to be treated with radiation. The prostate, a chestnut-sized organ, surrounds the neck of the bladder and urethra, the tube that carries urine out of the body. Surgery frequently caused complications that are not seen with radiation treatment.

Surgery was also once the usual treatment for cancer of the larynx, the voice box. Many patients found it difficult to learn a new way to talk, called esophageal speech, and artificial voice boxes weren't terribly satisfactory to many patients. Now radiation has largely replaced surgery and fewer patients lose their voice boxes to cancer.

Until recently, it was generally believed radiation was not an effective treatment for cancer of the rectum. "There used to be an old rule that said, if after radiation there was still tumour remaining at ninety days, the treatment had failed," explains one specialist. "Now we know response patterns differ in different kinds of cancer." Rectal cancer responds slowly. "When people realize there is an option and that the chances of success of surgery or radiation are about fifty-fifty, they often go for radiation," says the specialist.

"If the radiation works, they've kept their body intact. If it doesn't, we have surgery in reserve. The operation can still be done."

Early cancer of the ovary may be treated with radiation to the abdomen, following surgery. At Toronto's Princess Margaret Hospital, Canada's largest treatment centre, radiation is usually recommended, while in U.S. centres, chemotherapy is more common.

For leukemia patients, although chemotherapy is used to treat the diseased blood cells, radiation may be required to prevent the cancer from affecting the central nervous system.

Some leukemia patients are treated with bone marrow transplants. Bone marrow is the tissue in which blood cells originate. Radiation is used to destroy the patient's malignant cells before the healthy bone marrow cells are given to them. The largest number of bone marrow transplants performed in Canada are done at Princess Margaret Hospital which performs them at the rate of about one every ten days. In the United States, Seattle is well known as a bone marrow transplant centre because of the pioneering work of Dr. Donnell Thomas.

Although radiation is an effective weapon against cancer, it cannot be used against all kinds. Sometimes it can't be given because of the location of the tumour and sometimes because the kind of cells in the tumour are known to resist the impact of x-rays. For some patients radiation keeps cancer under control, although they cannot be cured, and they will require repeat treatment periodically. By shrinking tumours, radiation may also relieve pain that occurs when tumours press on nerves or block passageways.

"A lot of cancer can never be cured, it is a chronic disease," says one prominent radiation oncologist. "But it may not matter whether it is cured as long as the patient can function and live life more or less normally."

Some people are frightened of the side effects of radiation. They have many questions about what to expect. But people vary so much in the way their bodies react, it may be almost impossible to predict side effects. Certain people suffer none at all. It can depend on which part of the body is the target.

While radiation hits hardest the cells that are reproducing themselves, cancer cells are not the only cells doing that. Normal cells in the digestive tract reproduce themselves frequently and may be affected, causing some patients to feel nausea. Hair cells are also regularly replacing themselves and there may be hair loss.

Sometimes nurses and doctors are reluctant to tell you of possible side effects when you might not have them at all. But one study found that people who weren't warned felt angry and disappointed they hadn't been told in advance about side effects that did occur. On the other hand, those given information beforehand did not complain when no side effects materialized. They didn't think being told of adverse effects they might experience had caused them needless anxiety.

A number of patients feel fatigue after the first few treatments, with the weariness increasing after about eight sessions. Fatigue doesn't mean you are getting worse. You feel it because the body is using up much energy to restore normal cells that were damaged.

Some people feel pain after a few treatments. Destruction of the tumour may cause swelling that is painful. It will ease as the treatment continues and the tumour shrivels. Anti-pain and anti-nausea medications may help and you should ask your nurse or doctor about them if you feel you need them.

People who suffer no adverse effects occasionally worry that it means the treatment isn't working. Whether or not a person experiences side effects has no bearing on the effectiveness of the treatment.

Usually, there are no restrictions on the activities of patients during the course of treatment. You may be cautioned against driving yourself to the treatment centre because afterwards you may be too sleepy to drive safely home. Commonly, patients find they need extra rest. One nurse advises patients: "Listen to your body and if the message it is sending is to lie down, do it. Extra rest helps speed the recovery of normal tissue." Proper diet and drinking more fluid is also important. (See section on nutrition.)

You may find that as long as you don't push yourself too hard, you can work in your office, play golf, go to a movie, make love or whatever else you were doing before cancer so rudely interrupted.

Chemotherapy

When cancer cells have moved away from the tumour site or when cancer is all through the blood stream, as in leukemia, a weapon is needed against them that can travel through the whole body. Drugs can.

Since the late 1940s, a concerted scientific search has been under way for cancer drugs. Thousands of substances have been investigated and so far about fifty drugs have been proven useful. Cancer drugs aren't like drugs used to combat most other diseases. They are intended to kill human cells, not a bacteria or germ that has slipped into the body from outside. As the comic strip character Pogo once said: "We has seen the enemy and it is us." He could have been speaking of cancer. Cancer cells "is us."

The dream of cancer scientists has always been to find a "magic bullet"—a substance that would shoot down only cancer cells, sparing normal ones. But the big obstacle to such a discovery is that cancer cells are too much like normal cells. Chemical "bullets" that kill one, also kill the other.

But there is one vital difference. Cancer cells keep reproducing themselves. It means they require building materials and they need to be able to copy their genetic material to pass on to new cells.

Around 1950, a Boston doctor Sidney Farber, observed that children with leukemia got worse if they were given a vitamin, folic acid, which cells need. Without it, they die. It led Dr. Farber to create a drug, disguised as the vitamin, but which is really useless to a cell.

Cancer cells busily gathering nutrients pull in the drug mistaking it for the vitamin they need in order to live. The mistake sounds their death knell. The drug is called methotrexate and is widely used today.

About the same time, in London, Canada, Dr. Robert Noble was investigating the periwinkle plant. From folk medicine it was known to have medical powers and it looked as if it might have some use against diabetes. Instead, out of Dr. Noble's research came a cancer drug, vinblastin. Now it has two chemical cousins, vincristine and vindesine, that are also effective against cancer. They latch onto vital proteins in cells needed for cell reproduction, butting into the process and stopping it.

Doctors divide anti-tumour drugs into six categories. One group, alkylating agents, was developed from wartime studies of mustard gases. When one cell splits into two, it separates the two strands of genetic material so each can be copied. Alkylating agents hold the two strands together, interfering with reproduction.

Methotrexate is an example of the second group, called antimetabolites. They deprive growing cells of building materials. Others you may hear about in this group are ARA-C, which came from studies of ocean sponges and 5FU, which acts like a bad brick a cancer cell uses in constructing a new strand of genetic material. It ruins the new strand.

The third group is composed of special antibiotics. They come from bacteria. One of the most widely used is adriamycin. It gets between the strands of the genetic material to prevent the copying process. Another, bleomycin, is a mixture of substances produced by tiny organisms found in soil. It snips strands of genetic material into pieces.

The vincristine family, mentioned earlier, are known as alkaloids. The other two groups are hormones and miscellaneous compounds. Some tumour cells thrive on hormones and doctors can throw a tumour a nasty curve by supplying phony hormones or by depriving the cells of real hormones. Among the miscellaneous compounds, cisplatin, which is relatively new but is widely used, has proven particularly effective against cancer of the testicles and is a key reason for great advances in treatment of this cancer.

If you are to receive chemotherapy you will probably receive drugs from one or more of these groups. A combination of drugs is the usual strategy.

When the first successes with chemotherapy began to be reported, it gave little encouragement to the majority of cancer patients. Only rare cancers seemed to be cured by drugs. Burkitt's lymphoma, for example, was found to be curable with a single dose of an alkylating agent called cyclophosphamide. Burkitt's lymphoma, a cancer that starts in a child's jaw and spreads rapidly, occurs infrequently in North America although it is common in Africa.

But a single drug against the most common of childhood cancers, acute lymphocytic leukemia (ALL), brought discouraging results.

Gradually, doctors learned a single drug was not enough. To combat ALL took a combination of drugs. Before the chemotherapy was developed, the outlook for a child with ALL was bleak. Virtually none lived a normal life span and the majority died in a short time. Today 55 of 100 patients have a normal life expectancy. Some people who had ALL as children have already lived fifteen to twenty years free of disease and a number of them have had healthy children of their own.

Why will a combination of drugs work when a single drug does not? Doctors now know that as a cancer progresses, the cells develop a capacity to change. Although it began in one cell, a tumour is usually composed of a mixture of cell types by the time it is detected. A mixture of drugs may destroy a mixture of cells when a single drug couldn't get at all cell types.

The most dramatic achievement so far has been treatment of advanced Hodgkin's disease with a combination of drugs. Before 1963, Hodgkin's disease in advanced stages was incurable. Radiation was often effective in early cases but not in advanced ones. Now, by teaming up four drugs in a regime known as MOPP (each letter stands for a drug), doctors have a treatment that erases the disease in well over half the patients. MOPP was devised by Dr. Vincent DeVita of the U.S. National Cancer Institute.

With some patients disease-free for more than fifteen years, this might truly be considered a cure for many patients.

Doctors cannot stop drugs from damaging some normal cells but they have learned how to "rescue" normal cells with antidotes to the drugs, allowing them to give much larger doses of a drug to people with some kinds of cancer. For example, doctors can give doses of methotrexate a thousand times larger if it is followed by another drug, citrovorum factor, the antidote that rescues normal cells. Without the rescue, the large dose of methotrexate would be deadly.

A combination of chemotherapy, surgery and radiation is sometimes the most effective treatment. In a childhood cancer, Wilms' tumour, nine out of ten children are cured today by the three-pronged treatment. Previously only four in ten were freed of disease when surgery and radiation, but not drugs, were used.

Drug therapy after surgery for breast cancer that has spread beyond the breast is showing it can sharply reduce the risk of relapse and metastases. Surgery and radiation rid the women of cancer in breast and lymph nodes and no disease can be detected in their bodies, yet doctors know some of the women will have a recurrence of cancer. Chemotherapy may prevent it. Using drugs against invisible disease is called adjuvant therapy. It poses a dilemma because, in effect, it is designed to treat disease that nobody can be sure is there. Doctors know that in any given group of breast cancer patients, some harbour undetectable cancer cells and some do not. But they cannot tell which are which.

If cancer drugs were not so toxic it would be sensible to give them to all the patients just in case. But they are hard on the body. It is one thing to give them to a woman who unquestionably has cancer, but quite another when there is no evidence of cancer.

What should the doctor treating such a patient do? A panel of specialists from across the United States, after thoroughly reviewing the situation in 1980, concluded that because there is no definitive answer there must be frank and open discussion between physician and patient to make the patient fully aware of the dilemma and of both the benefits and hazards of accepting or rejecting adjuvant therapy. If you are facing this decision, be sure your doctor tells you as much as he or she can to help you understand.

So far, a number of studies indicate adjuvant therapy may be well worthwhile for young, pre-menopausal women with breast cancer that had spread to lymph nodes. It is less clear whether it is as useful for older women. However, more information continues to be gathered and in the near future there may be ways to track down undetected cancer cells using monoclonal antibodies. (See research section.)

Because many kinds of combination drug therapy have been developed so recently, not enough time has passed for long-term outcomes to be known. A number of doctors believe chemotherapy today is bringing about more cures than we yet realize. For example, fifteen years ago one kind of lung cancer, called small cell carcinoma, killed virtually all of its victims in a matter of weeks. Now, combination chemotherapy has freed of disease more than a quarter of the patients who were treated two to five years ago and it seems probable at least some of them will remain cancer-free and live a normal life span.

If you are to receive chemotherapy, your treatment will be planned and given under the supervision of a medical oncologist or by a blood specialist (hematologist). Where you receive the treatment depends on the drugs being used and how they are administered. It may be in a hospital or hospital clinic, the doctor's office, or at home.

Drugs may be given by mouth in the form of pills or drinks, be injected into a vein or muscle, dripped into a vein, or by tiny pumps or micro-capsules injected into the bloodstream. Small implantable pumps provide one of the newest ways of getting drugs to a tumour in steady doses. Placed so that they pump medication into a blood vessel leading to the tumour, they get stronger doses into the tumour site. Liver cancer is sometimes treated this way. The pump is implanted in the abdomen. Because the liver is the organ that deals with toxic substances in the body and neutralizes them, doctors think by putting the drugs more directly into the liver, the rest of the body may be spared from unwanted drug effects.

Micro-capsules that contain drugs also provide a new delivery system. The tiny containers are about the size of sugar grains. In the filtering system of the body, particles of certain sizes are trapped at particular locations. By adjusting the size of a micro-capsule, doctors can send in drugs that will be lodged at a particular site. Once caught, the capsule stays there while its contents leak out slowly, keeping a steady concentration of drugs aimed at the tumour. Your doctor will need to know whether you take medications of any kinds, including headache tablets, birth control bills, cough medicines or nose sprays. Some people don't think to mention items like these familiar products when they are asked about drugs they take. Your doctor will advise you whether or not you can continue to use regular medicines while you are receiving chemotherapy. Sometimes there are good reasons you should not do so.

There is no denying that chemotherapy may be tough on you. However, many patients sail through it with few or no adverse effects. Individual reactions vary widely. There is no relationship between how good or bad a person feels during treatment and the effectiveness of the treatment.

Drugs are designed to be gobbled by cells that are reproducing. Because cancer cells divide in two frequently, more of them take up the drugs than do normal cells which are likely to be in a resting stage. But some normal cells must replace themselves often and may be affected. They include hair follicles, cells in mouth, digestive tract, skin, bone marrow and reproductive organs. That is why side effects may include hair loss, stomach upsets, sore mouths or a drop in blood count.

You may feel your whole body equilibrium has gone topsy-turvy. Your emotions may roller-coaster. If so, try to remember these effects are often caused by cancer drugs. Some people, who have just come to terms with their disease and are feeling less emotional turmoil, fear they have again lost control. It may help to understand that the drugs are responsible.

Drugs can also cause muscle weakness and rashes, or make hands and feet fall asleep. This may sound like an endless list of side effects, but not all patients have all of them. You may not feel miserable or be bothered in any way. But if you are, keep in mind it is temporary. Almost always when a course of treatment is completed, normal well-being returns, skin clears, hair grows back and emotions settle down.

How long chemotherapy takes depends on the kind of cancer and the type of drugs. Some drugs cause changes in urine. Unless you are told in advance, you may be alarmed to find your urine is an unusual colour. Adriamycin makes urine red and methotrexate turns it bright yellow. Urine may have a strong medicinal smell. There is no reason to worry about these changes.

You will feel tired. The body is working hard to repair damage and is using much energy. Heed its message and get extra rest. If you are accustomed to an active life you will probably need to slow the pace and to allow yourself time to lie down during the day. Chemotherapy can also affect appetite. Some people don't feel like eating while others who formerly ate like sparrows feel ravenous. You can help your body recover strength by eating a well-balanced diet. (See section on nutrition.) You will need extra fluids to help your kidneys flush out the drugs. Particularly on days you receive your medications, you should drink eight to ten glasses of water, juice, tea or broth. Ask your doctor or nurse before using alcoholic beverages. It may be okay, but in some cases alcohol can interfere with chemotherapy.

Check with your doctor or nurse if you have any adverse reactions that worry you. They can help control major problems, such as nausea and pain if they occur, but nothing is too trivial to bring to their attention if it is troubling you.

If you dread the idea of hair loss, inquire about methods of cooling the head during treatment. Some research suggests that keeping hair follicles cooled temporarily stops them from reproducing. Putting them into a resting stage while the drugs are acting on cells may protect hair follicles. You can also help protect your hair by avoiding heat from hair dryers, electric rollers or curlers. Brush it gently with a baby brush or other soft-bristled brush. Don't put it in tight braids or corn-rows. Some people think a satin pillowcase to reduce friction is helpful. Don't have your hair coloured or permed. The chemicals may damage fragile hair. Use gentle products for shampooing. Covering your head with a wig or hat will not interfere with hair growth, contrary to the belief of some people who may tell you it will.

Before treatment begins, a dental check-up is usually recommended. It is particularly important for people who are to undergo therapy for leukemia, head and neck cancers, or who are receiving drugs that lower blood counts. Treatment may cause poor healing and any teeth that need to be extracted should come out before therapy begins. Mouth infections or abscesses also need attention prior to treatment.

Hormonal Therapy

Hormones are chemicals naturally produced in the body that carry out a number of different chores. Sex hormones, for example, play a big part in making a man manly and a woman feminine and in the process of reproduction.

In some cancers, such as prostate and certain kinds of breast cancer, tumour cells may need hormones to thrive. About fifty years ago, it was found that the female hormone, estrogen, curbed the growth of prostate cancers. It wasn't ideal treatment. It caused unwanted feminization of men, including breast growth. Over the years it was discovered also to damage the heart. Modern treatment of advanced prostate cancer uses drugs to deprive tumour cells of male hormones rather than giving estrogen. Depriving the tumours puts the brakes on their growth.

Some, but not all breast cancers, can be kept from growing by shutting off their supply of estrogen. Estrogens are produced by the ovaries and they help initiate the menstrual cycle, play a role in breast development at puberty and trigger other hormones that prepare a woman's body for pregnancy and breast feeding. Because part of their normal job is to stimulate cell growth, they may spur the growth of certain tumours.

In the past, doctors sometimes removed the ovaries of a patient with advanced breast cancer, hoping that without estrogen the tumour would be unable to keep growing. But the doctors had no way of telling in advance if it would work. In post-menopausal women whose ovaries had ceased functioning, adrenal glands, which are also involved in the production of hormones, were sometimes removed.

Doctors took a big step forward when they learned how to tell before such operations were performed whether the surgery would be useful. Cells that want estrogen, it was discovered, have on their outer surfaces receptors, rather like microscopic catchers' mitts, especially designed to grab estrogen. It is now possible to do tests that reveal whether the cells of a tumour have these receptors. If they don't, removing a woman's ovaries or adrenal glands is pointless. The tumour is not using estrogen.

Furthermore, today we have anti-estrogens, drugs that may deprive a tumour that needs estrogen from getting it. They are sometimes used instead of ovary removal surgery. They fit the cells "mitts" as if they were estrogen and stop the receptors from catching the real hormone. Progesterone is another female hormone some tumour cells need. A test is available to find out if the cells have progesterone receptors.

Hormonal therapy is commonly given right after surgery for breast cancer. It may be given alone or in combination with chemotherapy.

As well as breast and prostate cancer, other cancers that may be treated with hormones include Hodgkin's disease, other lymphomas, leukemias, myelomas, kidney, uterine and thyroid cancers. Synthetic hormones are included in combination chemotherapy. One of the drugs in the combination chemotherapy, MOPP, so successful against Hodgkin's disease, is a hormone-like substance, Prednisone.

Immunotherapy

Much effort has been put into a search for ways to increase the body's own ability to fight cancer. The body's defence mechanism, the immune system, is believed to protect against cancer. Some doctors say we all have cells turning malignant periodically but we do not necessarily get cancer because most of the time our immune system spots the troublemakers and destroys them. Doctors also have reason to believe the immune system guards us against cancer because it is known that people with suppressed immune systems, such as those given drugs to prevent rejection of transplanted organs, are more likely to develop cancer.

What role the immune system plays in safeguarding us from cancer or why it sometimes fails to do so is not fully understood. It may be that cancer cells, because they are our own cells, are not recognized as enemies by the immune system. For many years, researchers have tried to find ways to make cancer cells visible to the immune system so they would be attacked. Some medical scientists have attempted to increase the activity of the immune system generally by injecting agents known to spur the immune system into action because they are mistaken for infectious organisms. It was hoped that immune cells tracking down these agents would find and kill cancer cells in the process.

Scientists have searched for tumour antigens, which are rather like name-tags tumour cells might wear to identify them. They have found tumour-associated tags, but not ones worn exclusively by tumour cells.

Some experiments are underway designed to educate immune system cells to recognize and attack cells wearing certain antigens.

However, so far, no generally accepted immunotherapy has been devised.

Hyperthermia

High temperatures have long been observed to have harsh effects on tumour cells. Doctors noticed that sometimes fever, caused by an infection, brought a temporary halt to tumour growth. Years ago a Scottish doctor tried to treat patients by heating their whole bodies, encasing them in molten wax. But temperatures high enough to kill cancer cells couldn't be reached without also killing the patient.

With new technology came a new interest in heat therapy called hyperthermia. Radiofrequency waves, microwaves, ultrasound and space suits offer new ways to get heat into tumours. Experimental methods are being tried in several countries, including Canada, the United States and Britain. Modern hyperthermia is still in its infancy but many scientists think it may have great potential. Not enough is known yet about achieving high temperatures within a tumour. A temperature of about 45 degrees C (113 degrees F) is required to put a tumour cell out of commission. But the body has a highly efficient cooling system that mitigates against high heat in tissues. It protects us from overheating and, ordinarily, is a very desirable mechanism. But it works against doctors seeking to heat up tumours. Tumour cells are more vulnerable to heat than normal cells because they often have poor circulation.

Some evidence indicates hyperthermia may work in combination with radiation or chemotherapy. Cells that are hot appear to have trouble mending themselves so cancer cells damaged by treatment might, when heated, be unable to make repairs to their genetic material. Much more investigation of hyperthermia is needed before its worth will be known. Currently, it is likely to be suggested only in cases where no other treatments have been able to bring cancer under control.

Fifteen
Research: The hope for the future

WHEN WILL THERE be cures for all cancer? Nobody in the world today can make even a wild guess. But there are scientists who predict we will understand cancer by the year 2,000. Understanding cancer is quite a different matter from curing it. Yet only a few years ago any scientist who made such a prediction would have been considered foolhardy, if not mad. Today that goal seems within reach and as one scientist says: "Understanding what has gone wrong in a cell's machinery is a prerequisite for fixing it."

Over the years, cancer research often seemed like an enormous maze, full of dead ends, disappointing detours and frustrating blind alleys. Now researchers believe they are on a path through the thicket that truly leads to an explanation of cancer. From the scientists' point of view, the pace of advance has been fast and exciting in recent years. It may not seem so to people seeking answers today. The new findings that so elate cancer scientists may leave us scratching our heads in bewilderment. What on earth are oncogenes and monoclonal antibodies and recombinant DNA? What use are they to a cancer patient?

To put it in the simplest way possible, oncogenes are the segments of a cell's genetic material that go wrong and trigger cancer, monoclonal antibodies may be able to track down cancer cells anywhere in the body and recombinant DNA may be the technique by which cells gone wrong can be reprogrammed. Right now recombinant DNA allows scientists to probe the genetic material of cells so they can understand cancer.

169

Only a few years ago, scientists had no idea how a normal cell turned into a cancer cell. They suspected something had gone awry in the genetic instructions that guide cell processes. But until the 1970s, they had no way of finding out exactly what it was. The task was formidable. Your body contains some one hundred trillion cells, each housing tightly wound thread-like DNA (deoxyribonucleic acid), which if stretched out with pieces laid end to end would reach from here to the sun and back four hundred times. A cell's genetic material is made of DNA. It might be compared to a tape on which thousands of songs are recorded, with each song a gene. In each cell are up to 100,000 genes and each gene instructs the cell to make a particular protein whenever it is played. Also on the DNA tape are switches that turn a gene on when its protein is needed or off when it is not required.

The discovery that made it possible for researchers to investigate what individual genes do was the identification of a group of chemicals (enzymes) which can cut and patch strands of DNA. Cells use them to make repairs to DNA. With these enzymes, scientists could cut out a segment of DNA from a cell and splice it into the DNA of some other cell or bacterium. They could then observe what the second cell produced that it did not make before. Hence, they could learn what that particular segment (or gene) was for. Splicing a bit of DNA from one cell into another is recombinant DNA. (This technique has been used to produce human interferon in bacteria. Genes from human cells order the bacteria to produce the interferon, a natural body substance that may help combat certain cancers. Interferon research is described later.)

As scientists investigated human genes, putting them into animal cells to determine which human proteins the genes were for, something surprising happened. The astonishing discovery was that sometimes certain genes from human cells caused the animal cells to become cancer cells.

These genes were not rare. We all have them and so do all other kinds of life from fruit flies to tigers. It seemed incredible but we all carry genes that can cause cancer. Yet within a couple of years, scientists had found about thirty different kinds. These are the genes now called oncogenes or cancer genes, although scientists often say "pre-oncogene," meaning they have the potential to cause cancer although they may not have done so.

If we all have them, why don't we all have cancer? Researchers scrambled to find answers and it appears there may be several possible reasons.

Because oncogenes are so widespread in nature, it is probable they are essential to life. Some of them, it appears, play an important role before birth when a foetus is growing rapidly. They may not be intended to be switched on again in adulthood. Yet in some cancer cells they *are* turned on. Other oncogenes may be needed periodically throughout life and should shut on and off as required. But in cancer cells they may be stuck in the "on" position.

The next step was for researchers to discover what substances oncogenes order cells to make. Not surprisingly, at least some of them instruct cells to make proteins that are growth factors. The body has many different growth factors needed for wound healing or when cells must reproduce themselves to replace worn-out ones. Growth factors fit into chemical receptors on the surfaces of cells like keys fit locks. When they are inserted into the receptors, it is like turning on a car ignition. Inside the cell, it is as if a motor starts up and the cell begins the process of dividing. In normal cells, division stops when the replacement of tissue is complete. But among cancer cells, reproduction continues relentlessly. Why?

It may be there is a slight error in the gene's DNA. Researchers at the Massachusetts Institute of Technology, Boston, led by Dr. Robert Weinberg, found an oncogene taken from a bladder cancer cell varied in one tiny way when it was compared with the same gene taken from a normal cell. Among the 6,000 chemical units that form the gene, one was different. Subsequently, similar tiny differences have been found in oncogenes from lung cancer cells.

In other cases, an oncogene may have lost its off switch or come under the control of a wrong switch that turns it on too often. Genes are strung along 46 chromosomes and often in tumour

172 / *Understanding Cancer*

cells, pieces of chromosome are missing or pieces have broken off the chromosome to which they belong and hooked onto some other chromosome. Genes in the wrong place might be turned on when they shouldn't be.

With the possibility of such tiny errors in DNA or misplaced pieces of it leading to cancer, it seems astonishing that trillions of cells in our body remain normal. But now it is known one oncogene alone does not make a healthy cell malignant. British and American scientists have found it takes at least two genetic changes. One change may prime the cell but unless a second oncogene gets in the act, cancer does not occur. The changes might happen years apart. They might be brought about by exposure to chemicals or radiation from the environment or substances in the diet. You can see why discovering the cause of cancer is so complex.

Over the years of our lives, our DNA is repeatedly being broken or damaged. But we have built-in repair mechanisms and in human cells these mechanisms are remarkably good. One of the discoverers of DNA repair processes, Malcolm Patterson of Canada's Chalk River Nuclear Laboratories, has said were it not for our cellular repair crews, the enzymes that cut and patch DNA, the incidence of cancer would be so great life as we know it would probably be impossible.

People with defective repair mechanisms are at high risk of cancer. Much research in Canada and other countries is under way to study genes that direct DNA repair. The aim is to find out how to protect those people who are prone to cancer and from them to learn what might be done to protect everybody.

It is not expected that research into genes can hope to be translated into new treatments in the immediate future. The inner workings of cells and the interaction between cells are unbelievably complex. Researchers have a long way to go. Yet they have today, as they never had before, the ability to delve into the origins of cancer.

At the same time, other research is already pushing monoclonal antibodies from the laboratory to treatment and diagnostic centres. Studies using these special antibodies began following the discovery in 1975 in Britain, of how to make them. The brainchild of George Kohler and Cesar Milstein, in Cambridge, the antibodies were like booster rockets to research. The two scientists found a way to produce in the laboratory, in unlimited quantities, any specific antibody that might be required.

Antibodies are special proteins that act like tracking dogs trained to search out a quarry. In our bodies, antibodies are produced by cells of the immune system called B-cells. We make many different kinds because each is tailored to fit a particular molecule called an antigen. For example, if a measle virus infected you, your B-cells would produce an army of antibodies that precisely fit an antigen on the virus. These antibodies would track down measle viruses and clamp onto the antigen.

If a doctor wanted to find out if you had measles, he could take a sample of blood and mix it with measle antibodies. If the measle virus was present, there would be clumps of antibody latched onto antigen, interlocked in antibody-antigen complexes. The diagnosis would be certain.

In scores of laboratories, scientists use this technique to search out differences between tumour cells and normal cells. Antibodies produced in the laboratory to latch onto tumour cell antigens, but ignore normal cells, would provide a method of finding metastatic cells and of delivering chemotherapy exclusively to the tumour. For diagnosis, radioactive materials could be attached to the antibodies which would light up like dots of light on a scan, showing doctors the tumour and any cells that had spread. For treatment, drugs could be attached to the antibodies to be carried only to cancer cells. In some cases the antibodies themselves might conquer cancer cells.

In 1981, one of the first cases in which monoclonal antibodies were used to treat a patient was reported in the New England Journal of Medicine. Researchers at Stanford Medical Center, California, created antibodies to certain cells of a 67-year-old man with a rare, virulent form of lymphoma. Over five weeks of treatment his disease disappeared. However, in general, monoclonal antibodies are expected to be more effective as carrier pigeons, transporting drugs to a tumour.

Antigens specific to tumour cells have been elusive, but the search for them continues. Scientists have found some associated with certain cancers, although not exclusively on cancer cells. One antibody associated with malignant melanoma has been attached to a plant toxin called ricin, derived from castor beans. Cells take up ricin, which then poisons them. The new treatment is being tested experimentally in some patients.

Ricin has also been linked to other monoclonal antibodies to treat bone marrow that is to be used for transplant. Unlike most transplants which may be attacked by white cells of the recipient's body, bone marrow contains the donor's white cells that may attack the patient. Cells in the donor bone marrow that would do this can now be identified by antibodies and poisoned by ricin before the marrow is injected into the patient. Not only is rejection prevented but it is beginning to make possible a bone marrow transplant from a donor who is not a blood relative of the patient. Previously, the donor had to be a close relative, preferably brother or sister, whose tissue matched the tissue of the patient.

Other research involves drugs that spring into action when they are exposed to light. This new kind of drug treatment is called photodynamic therapy. It works this way: the drugs are put into the body at the site of the tumour and are taken up by both cancer and normal tissues. However, they do not begin acting until they are exposed to red light. Normal cells rid themselves of the drug in a short time but it stays in tumour cells longer. Doctors wait until the normal cells have been cleared of the drug and then apply the light. The drug goes to work against tumour cells. The molecules of the drugs are large and stay in tumour cells longer because tumour cells, characteristically, have poor drainage systems.

This new treatment was first used in Japan for lung cancer and doctors reported the first patient was still free of disease three years later. Now it has shown to be a promising therapy for bladder cancer. It can be used in conjunction with radiation and other chemotherapy.

Research is under way in several countries, including Canada and the United States, to learn the most effective ways of giving this fascinating new type of therapy.

Products naturally produced in the body to combat illness, of which interferon is one, comprise another group of substances under study. There are three kinds of interferon being investigated. For a time, hopes soared that interferon would prove to be highly effective. It is still being extensively studied but is has fallen back to a relatively low position in the ranks of anti-cancer weapons. Nevertheless, there have been enough good responses to interferon among some cancer patients to be tantalizing. Doctors are also finding a way to spur the body's own production of interferon. Interferon plays a role in combating viruses, so doctors can coax the body to produce it by injecting drugs that are actually artificial viruses. Scientists do not yet fully understand how interferon works in the body but it is known that when a person has a virus infection, like a common cold, interferon escapes from infected cells and warns other cells to man battle stations and protect themselves.

When it is given to patients, interferon makes many of them feel as if they have the flu, with chills, aches, fever and muddled thinking. But the symptoms clear up fairly quickly. Some studies indicate interferon may turn out to be most useful in concert with cancer drugs, boosting drug effectiveness. But other studies have raised alarm by suggesting that sometimes interferon seems to increase the spread of cancer or cause heart problems.

Other proteins formed naturally in the body, which like interferon play a role in the immune mechanism, are also being studied. One, called interleukin, seems to crank up defence activity. The body appears to have a stack of such protective weapons and so far research has only scratched the surface of understanding this built-in armament.

The immune system is marvellously intricate. As well as B-cells which produce antibodies, it has platoons of T-cells that keep watch for any cells in the body that do not belong there. T-cells tell your body what is you and what is not you. If you had a kidney transplant, your T-cells would know the kidney you were given wasn't really you. Unless they were subdued by drugs, they would attack and reject the transplant.

In 1984, cancer researchers in Toronto and California simultaneously discovered a gene in T-cells that enable these cells to distinguish alien cells from self. With orders from the gene, the cell manufactures a receptor on the surface of the cell by which it detects the difference.

The discovery immediately gave doctors a better way to distinguish one kind of leukemia from another, by showing whether the sick white cells were B-cells or T-cells. Those with the receptors, of course, were T-cells. Monoclonal antibodies tailored to fit the receptors could pick out T-cells. Leukemic cells are often so immature and abnormal it is difficult to tell what kind of white cells they are. It is important to know in order to plan the best treatment.

Discovery of the T-cell receptor also opened the door to an explosion of new studies that may help explain why cancer cells are not always recognized as enemy cells and destroyed by the immune system. It seems strange that the eye, with the aid of a microscope, can see obvious difference between orderly rows of normal cells and haphazard lumps of cancer tissue, yet the immune system is not always able to notice the bizarre looking cancer cells. Research into the T-cell receptor to learn how it recognizes alien cells holds the promise of tagging cancer cells so T-cells will attack and kill them.

The most insidious thing about cancer is its ability to spread. If it stayed put, cancer would rarely cause death. In recent years, researchers have found out much about how tumour cells metastasize. Not all the cells of a tumour are able to do it. But the small number that can are able to stick themselves to a protein called laminin. Laminin is found in membranes that separate different tissues rather like living fences. When a tumour cell attaches itself to laminin, it releases enzymes that chop the fence, causing it to fall apart and let the tumour cell through. Now scientists are finding ways of keeping the fence intact to block the spread of cancer.

Tumour cells that leave the main tumour seem to know where they should go. Some are directed specifically to the liver, for example, or to bone. Doctors call it organ specific metastasis. Researchers are studying molecules on tumour cells that tell them when they have reached their new home. The molecules clasp onto cells at the new site, in effect dropping anchor so they can stay there to start a new tumour. In future it may be possible to prevent tumour cells from settling at new sites. Ways may be found to interfere with the anchorage molecules.

Many tumour cells never make it to their new homesites. They die *en route*. Blood cells can squeeze through very narrow blood vessels changing from spheres to sausage-like shapes. Most cancer cells cannot do that and they perish trying to get through tiny capillaries. But some do manage the trip successfully. Scientists are investigating the ways cells of a tumour differ from each other. In future, treatment may be designed to kill tumour cells that can travel. It has been estimated that if metastases can be stopped, 90 per cent of cancers will be curable. "If we're going to treat metastases successfully, we must get around the problem of cell diversity — between the primary tumour and its metastases and among the metastases themselves," explains one researcher. tases successfully, we must get around the problem of cell diversity — between the primary tumour and its metastases and among the metastases themselves," explains one researcher.

It has been only in recent years that scientists have realized a tumour is usually made up of a mixture of cells. As a tumour grows, its cells differentiate (change to different types). The cells may look alike under the microscope but they do not all behave alike.

That is why a combination of drugs or radiation used with drugs frequently provides more effective treatment than a single agent. Doctors now use computerized programmes to simulate different drug strategies and predict the most effective combination of drugs, doses and timing of treatment. One of the first such programmes was devised by Dr. James Goldie of the Cancer Control Agency, British Columbia.

Dr. Goldie says tumour cells that are resistant to drugs occur at random, as the cancer cells differentiate. A tumour is curable if it is treated before resistant cells are created. That is why doctors need to know the combinations of drugs that will kill all types of cells in the tumour before drug-resistant cells develop.

Much research is aimed at finding new drugs or improving

old ones. The goal is to discover products that are easier on patients yet harder on tumours. This is one area of research in which patients take part.

Once new drugs have been shown to have anti-cancer effects on mice in which human tumours are grown and in tumour cells growing in dishes of nutrients in the laboratory, the next step is to test them on patients in a clinical trial. Roughly, one in every 5,000 compounds investigated seems worthy of going to clinical trial.They are tried first in large animals, dogs or monkeys, to see if they are safe to use. Even so, it cannot be known how toxic they will be to people until volunteers try them.

New drugs are tested in a four-stage process. The Phase I study is concerned with determining a safe dose. It is often difficult for patients and their families to understand Phase I studies. A patient may be able to accept the fact that doctors cannot promise a new drug will work, but patients do expect their physicians to know how much of the drug to give them. Yet at this point in drug research, the size of a safe and tolerable dose is not known. Ordinarily, a patient receives a low dose to start and the dosage is gradually increased to the point where toxic effects are observed.

Usually, only a small number of people take part in Phase I studies. They are people with severe disease for which there is no known effective treatment. For the patients there is a chance of a long shot that the new drug might work for them when nothing else can. But it is a gamble. People who take part in such studies must be fully informed that the treatment offers them slim hope but it may help future patients. Doctors conducting such trials need finely-honed skills to ensure as little harm as possible comes to patients, in the process of determining the size of doses safe to use.

The Declaration of Helsinki states: "Clinical research cannot legitimately be carried out unless the importance of the objective is in proportion to the inherent risk to the subject."

Patients and doctors, in the past, have believed the objective was worth a risky venture into the unknown. Had they not, we would not have the successful treatments for cancer that exist today. But for a person to agree to take part in such a study is never a simple decision and he or she is entitled to the fullest information possible.

When safe doses of a new drug have been determined, the compound moves on to a Phase II trial. It is given to groups of patients with different kinds of cancer. It is tested against a variety of cancers because some drugs work well against certain tumours but not against others. At this stage, doctors still cannot tell patients that there is a good chance the drug will work. It is simply not known how effective it will be. Phase II studies are designed to study the effectiveness of the new substance in shrinking tumours and prolonging life. As in Phase I, patients who take part are those who cannot be helped by any known treatment.

When a drug has made it through these first two phases and has shown itself to be safe and effective, it still remains to be seen how it stacks up against treatments already in use. In Phase III, matched patients with similar tumours are given parallel treatment. Half will follow the new drug route, half the old treatment regime and the outcomes are compared. If the new substance is as good or better, it is approved for wider use.

Commonly, in trials comparing treatments, patients are "randomized" — that is, patients are selected at random as to who will be given which treatment. It puts doctors in a prickly situation. Many patients want their doctors to tell them the best treatment, not to have the treatment selected out of a hat. Yet, in all honesty, the doctor doesn't know which is best. The new treatment may turn out to be far superior. It may not. Only after many cases are compared will the answer be learned.

While Phase I seeks to answer the question *Is it safe?* and Phase II the question *Is it effective?* Phase III studies seek to learn how well it works. Patients taking part in this third level of testing at least can be reassured the treatment has been effective in some other patients.

Scientists who discover new treatments deserve credit, but patients who take part in clinical trials are equally deserving. They are a very special breed of selfless pioneers.

In the final phase, the new drug is approved for use by doctors in many centres so responses and side effects can be monitored in a large number of patients.

Not all research involving patients deals with drugs or other treatments. Studies gaining momentum in recent years are also concerned with diet and nutrition. Through interviews with patients and their families, researchers are looking into the eating habits of patients and comparing their life-long food patterns with those of people, matched in age, sex and environment, who do not get cancer. From these studies, researchers have gathered some evidence that suggests fresh vegetables and fruits eaten daily and diets moderate in fat reduce the risk of cancer.

In the future, we may know how to protect ourselves from some kinds of cancer by eating an anti-cancer diet. It is already known from research how some small amounts of trace metals or selenium help in protecting or repairing DNA of normal cells. Vitamin C, discovered in 1932 by Dr. Albert Szent-Georgyi, in the United States, has been shown to protect cells by soaking up certain particles that may crash around inside cells like bulls in a china shop causing cell damage. Vitamin E captures substances that can damage cell membranes.

But research has also shown that too much of a good thing can do harm. High doses of Vitamin C, for instance, have been found to aid tumour growth in rats and guinea pigs. Too much selenium or overdoses of Vitamin A are poisonous.

The day may come when, with a quick lab test, the level of a person's protection against cancer will be measured and if it needs tuning up, the doctor will prescribe a change in diet.

Other studies underway are intended to determine whether certain foods can help stop cancer in its tracks after it has developed. Long-range studies in Toronto by Dr. Robert Bruce of the Ludwig Cancer Institute involve the use of vitamins, calcium, and fibre against cancer.

In another realm of research, patients are taking part in studies concerned with the quality of life. Saving life isn't enough if it leaves a person sentenced to a wretched existence or emotionally crippled by fear and depression.

Scientists in the field of human values research are finding out how people adapt to life-threatening illness and learning that a number of patients are able to turn a potentially tragic blow into a benefit. In one study with 78 breast cancer patients, psychologists found 53 per cent reported they had experienced only positive results in their lives as a result of their disease. "When you consider that these women usually had disfiguring surgery, had often had painful follow-up care and had been seriously frightened and lived under the shadow of possible recurrence, this is a remarkable ability to construe personal benefit from potential tragedy," one of the researchers reported.

Among the good changes the women described were deeper self-knowledge, a sharper awareness of pleasure and discovering which things in life were most important. "I feel as if I were for the first time really conscious," said one woman. "I have much more enjoyment each day, each moment. I am not so worried about what is or isn't or what I wish I had." Another said, "You take a long look at your life and realize that many things you thought were important before are totally insignificant."

By learning how patients like these direct their thinking and feelings to come to the conclusion their lives are better because of cancer, social scientists hope to develop strategies to help other people, not only cancer patients, but anyone who has been emotionally shattered.

It may not be possible to cure all cancer in the foreseeable future, but there is a high probability the percentage of people whose lives can be saved will continue to increase steadily and that people living with chronic cancer will be assured of being able to have lives that are satisfying and productive. The myth of cancer will be a thing of the past.

Glossary

Some words you hear that are related to cancer and its treatment may be new to you. Here is an alphabetical list to assist you:

Accelerator   machines such as a Betatron or linear accelerator that accelerate particles to high energies to create radiation therapy to treat tumours.

Adenocarcinoma   a malignant growth of epithelial cells in a gland-like pattern.

Adenine   one of four building blocks of DNA, the genetic material found in all cells. The other three are cytosine, guanine and thymine.

Adjuvant Chemotherapy   use of cancer drugs following surgery to ward off possible recurrence.

Adriamycin   anti-cancer drug that interferes with cell division.

Alopecia   hair loss.

Alpha-Fetoprotein   proteins found in embryonic tissues, usually absent in adults but which may reappear with onset of certain kinds of cancer.

Amino Acids   the main components of proteins.

Anemia   condition marked by low number of red blood cells.

Angiography   visualization of blood vessels by x-ray.

Angiosarcoma   malignant tumour originating in a blood vessel.

Antibody   protein formed by the body immune system; there are many kinds of antibody, each specific to an antigen.

Antigen   molecule, frequently protein, of a cell or other living organism like a virus, against which the immune system can make an antibody.

Antimetabolite   a fake nutrient used as a chemotherapy agent.

Antiserum   serum containing antibody.

Anorexia   severe loss of appetite.

Axilla   the armpit where axillary nodes are located beneath the shoulder.

Barium Enema   barium sulfate introduced into the intestinal tract to allow sharper x-ray examination of lower bowel.

Basal Cell Carcinoma common kind of skin cancer that forms in the lowermost layer of the skin.

Benign Tumour abnormal swelling or growth that is not cancer.

Betatron machine that accelerates electrons used for radiation therapy of deep tumours.

BCG tuberculosis immunization preparation used to stimulate the immune system for immunotherapy.

BCNU anti-cancer drug of alkylating agent drug group.

Biopsy removal of tissue from the living body to be examined microscopically to diagnose cancer.

Blood Count numbers of red cells, white cells, or platelets determined from a blood sample.

B-Lymphocytes kind of white cells originating in bone marrow that are part of the immune system.

Breast Self-Examination examining the breasts in a circular pattern to detect lumps or changes, a technique women are encouraged to learn and use regularly to monitor their own breasts.

Bone Marrow soft tissue in the centre of bones where blood is manufactured.

Burkitt's Lymphoma cancer affecting face region mostly found in African children.

Capillary a tiny blood vessel.

Carcinogen cancer-causing agent.

Carcinogenesis creation of cancer.

Carcinoma malignant tumour originating from epithelial tissue, which is tissue that covers or lines organs, glands and other body parts.

CEA carcinoembryonic antigen—protein material found in association with certain cancers and used for diagnostic blood test.

Cell Differentiation progressive diversification of cells as they become specialized.

Cervix neck or opening of the uterus (womb).

Chemotherapy treatment with anti-cancer drugs.

Choriocarcinoma cancer arising in part of the placenta, the organ that nourishes an unborn baby.

Clinical commonly used in "clinical trials" or "clinical research" to mean involving patients in study and research such as testing new cancer drugs or other treatments.

Cobalt-60 artificially produced isotope of cobalt that produces gamma rays used in radiation therapy.

Colon the part of the large intestine that extends from the end of the small intestine to the rectum.

Colonoscopy technique for examining the large bowel by means of a flexible tool called a colonoscope.

Colostomy surgical procedure which creates a new opening from the colon to body surface to permit elimination of body wastes.

Colposcopy examination of the vagina and cervix with a magnifying instrument, called a colposcope, to check for abnormal tissue.

Complement a group of proteins in the blood that form an important part of the immune system.

Complete Response total disappearance of a tumour.

Computed Tomography also called computerized axial tomography CAT scan or CT scan, a way of imaging the body using narrow beams of x-rays and a computer. "Tomos" comes from Greek word meaning to slice.

Cyclotron accelerator used to propel atomic particles to create radiation for therapy.

Cyst abnormal sac in the body containing liquid or semi-solid.

Cytotoxic toxic to cells, commonly used to indicate cell-killing chemotherapy.

DES dicthylstilbestrol, a synthetic female hormone found capable of causing cancer in the offspring of women who took it during pregnancy. Also used in treatment of some breast and prostate cancers.

Diagnostic Radiology imaging, such as by x-ray, to detect and identify disease.

DNA deoxyribonucleic acid, the genetic material that controls life processes.

Doppler Scanning technique used in ultrasound imaging to monitor movement such as the flow of blood.

Dosimetrist person responsible for planning and calculating radiation dose.

Electron negatively charged sub-atomic particle.

Electron Microscope optical instrument that uses a beam of electrons to produce an enlarged image on a screen; can magnify up to 300,000 times real size.

Endometrial having to do with the lining of the uterus (womb).

Endoscope instrument used to examine the interior of an organ such as the bladder.

Enterostomy Therapist health professional trained in the care of stomas, which are artificial openings into the body.

Enzyme compound produced in the body involved in chemical processes in cells; body makes many different kinds.

Epidemiology study of disease in populations.

Epithelial Tissue   covering or lining of parts of the body, including skin and organs.

Esophageal Speech   speech technique for people without voice boxes, accomplished by swallowing and expelling air from the esophagus (gullet).

Estrogen   female hormones, secreted by the ovaries.

Etiology   cause of disease.

Ewings Sarcoma   malignant tumour of bone, arising in the marrow.

Excision   surgical removal of piece of the body.

Experimental Models   usually refers to animal studies that serve to predict effects in man.

Five Year Survival   a benchmark in the evaluation of response to treatment.

Fluoroscopy   diagnostic imaging, converting x-rays into visible light to be displayed on a screen.

5-FU   5-fluorouracil, an anti-metabolite drug, used to treat several kinds of cancer.

Gamma Rays   radiation with wave length shorter than x-rays emitted by Cobalt-60 and radium, often called x-rays when emitted by a machine.

Gene   hereditary unit of life, a segment of DNA carrying the code for a specific protein.

Genetic Code   the sequence of amino acids in genetic material.

Genome   the entire genetic information carried by a cell.

Germ Cells   sperm cells and ova (egg), the cells involved in reproduction.

Giant Cell Sarcoma   tumour of bone containing many large cells which have many nuclei.

Guaiac Test   chemical test used to detect hidden blood in stool for diagnosis of colon-rectum cancer, or any other gastro-intestinal tract cancer, including stomach.

Hematocrit   blood test that determines the volume of red blood cells.

Hepatoma   liver tumour.

Hodgkin's Disease   form of cancer that affects the lymphatic system, distinguished from other lymphomas by the presence of a particular abnormal cell called Reed-Sternberg cell.

Hormone   chemical product of the endocrine glands that helps regulate body mechanisms; the body produces many kinds.

Hormonotherapy   treatment by use of hormones.

Hospice   programme or place of care, designed to meet range of needs of terminally ill patients and their families.

Hyperthermia   raising temperature of tissue as a method of treatment or to enhance other forms of treatment.

Hysterectomy   surgical procedure for removal of the uterus.

Ileostomy   surgical procedure to construct an artificial opening for small intestine to eliminate waste.

Image Intensifier   electronic device to present a bright image from x-rays generally displayed on TV-type screen.

Immunology   science concerned with the body's immune system which is the defence mechanism.

Immunotherapy   treatment by stimulating body defences against disease.

Incidence   number of cases of a specific disease occurring in a given population during a certain period of time.

Interstitial Therapy   radiotherapy in which needles, wires or seeds containing radioactive material are put directly into the body. Also called internal radiation.

Intravenous   put into the bloodstream through a vein.

Interferon   substances produced by the body to help combat virus infections, under study by cancer scientists and being tested as treatment.

In Situ   remaining at the site of origin.

Invasive   growing into adjacent tissue.

Jaundice   yellow discolouration of the skin and other tissue.

Kaposi's Sarcoma   kind of cancer previously rarely seen in younger people, but sometimes occurring in those stricken with AIDS, acquired immune deficiency syndrome.

Killer Cells   cells that are part of the immune system.

Laser   acronym for light amplification by stimulated emission of radiation, small beams of radiation intense enough to produce heat or vibration that can be used as a precise surgical tool.

Leukemia   cancer of blood forming tissue characterized by abnormal production of white cells. Acute lymphocytic leukemia, ALL, is the most common childhood cancer.

Leukocytes   white blood cells.

Linear Accelerator   device to accelerate electrons used in radiation therapy.

Lumpectomy   operation to remove a lump from the breast.

Lymph   nearly clear fluid circulating in the body, containing white cells called lymphocytes, antibodies and nourishing material.

Lymph Gland   also called lymph node, filters tissue fluid and produces some white blood cells called lymphocytes.

Lymphoma   malignant disease of lymph tissues.
Lymph System   a network of tissues that form a drainage system to carry fluid from cells and tissues.

Macrophage   type of white blood cell that engulfs and breaks down unwanted cells and acts as garbage collector.
Mammography   diagnostic x-ray examination of the breast.
Mastectomy   surgical removal of the breast.
Melanoma   cancer of pigment cells usually in the skin.
Metabolism   physical and chemical processes of living organism, that maintains it and creates its energy.
Metastasis   process by which cancer cells break away and spread to start up new tumours.
Mitosis   process of cell reproduction to make new cells.
Molecule   tiny mass of matter.
MOPP   combination of four drugs used in treatment of Hodgkin's disease.
Multiple Myeloma   cancer arising in bone marrow causing a proliferation of cells in blood plasma that release a protein that can be identified in blood. Destruction of bone is prime characteristic of this cancer.
Mutagen   substance which alters cell genetic material. Many mutagens are also cancer-causing agents.

Neoplasm   new abnormal growth, may be benign or malignant but more commonly used to denote malignant tumours.
Neuroblastoma   malignant tumour of the nervous system.
Nucleic Acid   DNA or RNA (ribonucleic acid) which exert control over life processes.
Nucleus   core of a cell containing chromosomes; some cells like red blood cells have no nucleus but most do.
Nuclear Magnetic Resonance   a technique for imaging internal structures and metabolic reactions of the body.
Nuclear Medicine   medical practice that makes use of radioactive materials for diagnostic studies.

Oncogenesis   creation of cancer.
Oncogenic   cancer-causing.
Oncology   the study of tumours, a special branch of medicine; an oncologist is a doctor who specializes in cancer therapy.
Oophorectomy   surgical removal of the ovaries.
Ostomy   surgical procedure to create a stoma, an artificial opening.
Osteogenic Sarcoma   tumour of bone.

Palliative   providing relief from pain and emotional and spiritual distress.

Palpation   feeling with the hands to detect abnormality or tumour.

Pap Test   test to detect cancer of the cervix by collecting cells from the vagina for microscopic study.

Pathogenic   capable of causing disease.

Phagocytosis   ingestion of particles by immune system cells.

Platelets   small circular discs in the blood necessary for stopping bleeding.

Plasma   liquid part of blood with cells removed.

Plasma Cell   type of white blood cell.

Pleural Effusion   fluid in chest.

Pneumonectomy   surgical procedure to remove an entire lung.

Polyp   a small growth, often benign.

Proctosigmoidoscopy   examination of rectum and lower colon with a tubular instrument.

Prognosis   a prediction as to the course and outcome of disease and the prospect for recovery.

Prosthesis   an artificial limb or any other part of the body, an artificial replacement.

Protocol   standardized procedures followed by doctors.

P.R.N.   prescription order meaning "as needed".

Quackery   the practice of fraudulent methods of therapy for which unjustified claims are made or of methods of treatment never shown to be effective.

Radiotherapy   treatment of disease by x-rays or other radiant energy.

Radiotherapist   a doctor specializing in treatment of cancer by radiation.

Radiologist   a doctor who specializes in diagnosing disease by using x-rays.

Regional Involvement   when cancer has spread from the original site to neighbouring areas.

Remission   complete or partial disappearance of symptoms and evidence of disease; also the period of time a disease is under control.

Residual Disease   cancer left behind following tumour removal.

Retinoblastoma   a cancer of the eye.

RNA   ribonucleic acid, the companion of DNA, in cells, which plays a part in the control of life processes.

Sarcoma   form of cancer arising in connective tissue, bones, cartilage and muscle.

Serum   the clear portion of body fluid, blood from which cells and other solids have been removed.

Sigmoid   the S-shaped part of the colon.

Sputum Test   study of cells from the lungs found in sputum that has been coughed up.
Staging   determining the extent or stage of a cancer.
Stomatitis   inflammation in the mouth, sometimes with sores.

Teletherapy   radiation therapy administered by an external beam from a machine.
Tissue Culture   laboratory cultivation of cells within a flask or dish.
Transformation   change in the appearance and behaviour of cells.
Tracheostomy   surgical procedure to create a permanent opening in the windpipe. A temporary opening is called a tracheotomy.
Thymus Gland   small gland near the heart involved in producing T-cells that are vital to the immune system.

Ultra-sound   high frequency sound used to image internal structures by bouncing back sound waves.
Unproven Methods   untested or dubious ways of treating cancer.
Urostomy   surgical procedure to create an opening to allow elimination of urine.

Virology   the science of studying viruses.
Virus   sub-microscopic agent that infects cells of humans, animals or plants and is unable to multiply outside living cells.

Wilms' Tumour   a cancer of the kidney, usually occuring early in childhood.
WBC count   white blood cell count, to assess the number of each kind of leukocyte (white blood cell).

Xeroradiography   a form of mammography.
X-Ray   radiations of short wave length, shorter than ultraviolet light, used to diagnose and treat cancer.

Zeugmatography   another name for NMR imaging or nuclear magnetic resonance.

Directory: Where to find help

Canadian Cancer Society: National
Office
130 Bloor St. West
Suite 1001
Toronto, Ontario
M5S 2V7
Telephone (416) 961-7223

American Cancer Society
777 Third Avenue
New York, N.Y. 10017
Telephone (212) 371-2900

Canada: Provincial Divisions of the Canadian Cancer Society

Alberta Division
Suite 310
2424-4th St. S.W.
Calgary, Alberta
T2S 2T4
Telephone (403) 228-4487

British Columbia and Yukon Division
955 West Broadway St.
Vancouver, British Columbia
V5Z 3X8
Telephone (604) 736-1211

Manitoba Division
777 Portage Ave., 2nd Floor,
Suite 202
Winnipeg, Manitoba
R3G 0N3
Telephone (204) 774-7483

New Brunswick Division
P.O. Box 2089
Saint John, New Brunswick
E2L 3T5
Telephone (506) 652-7600

Newfoundland Division
P.O. Box 8921
St. John's, Newfoundland
A1B 3R9
Telephone (709) 753-6520

Nova Scotia Division
201 Roy Building
1657 Barrington St.
Halifax, Nova Scotia
B3J 2A1
Telephone (902) 423-6183

Ontario Division
1639 Yonge St.
Toronto, Ontario
M4T 2W6
Telephone (416) 488-5400

Prince Edward Island Division
57 Queen St., 4th Floor
P.O. Box 115, Hyndman Bldg.
Charlottetown, Prince Edward
Island
C1A 7K2
Telephone (902) 894-9675

Quebec Division
1118 St. Catherine St. W.#700
Montreal, Quebec
H3B 1H5
Telephone (514) 866-1112

Saskatchewan Division
2629-29th Ave.
Regina, Saskatchewan
S4S 2Y9
Telephone (306) 584-1054

In Canada, your nearest Canadian Cancer Society unit or branch will provide information on these Canadian Cancer Society services:

CanSurmount
Coping with Cancer groups
Mastectomy Visiting Service
Lodge Accommodation

Consult your local telephone directory for the Cancer Society unit or branch in your community or contact the provincial division listed above.

U.S.A.: Chartered Divisions Of The American Cancer Society, Inc.

Alabama Division, Inc.
2926 Central Avenue
Birmingham, Alabama 35209
(205) 879-2242

Alaska Division, Inc.
1343 G. Street
Anchorage, Alaska 99501
(907) 277-8696

Arizona Division, Inc.
634 West Indian School Road
P.O. Box 33187
Phoenix, Arizona 85067
(602) 234-3266

Arkansas Division, Inc.
5520 West Markham Street
P.O. Box 3822
Little Rock, Arkansas 72203
(501) 664-3480-1-2

California Division, Inc.
1710 Webster Street
P.O. Box 2061
Oakland, California 94604
(415) 893-7900

Colorado Division, Inc.
2255 South Oneida
P.O. Box 24669
Denver, Colorado 80224
(303) 758-2030

Connecticut Division, Inc.
Bames Park South
14 Village Lane
P.O. Box 410
Wallingford, Connecticut 06492
(203) 265-7161

Delaware Division, Inc.
Academy of Medicine Bldg.
1708 Lovering Avenue
Suite 202
Wilmington, Delaware 19806
(302) 654-6267

District of Columbia Division, Inc.
Universal Building, South
1825 Connecticut Avenue, N.W.
Washington, D.C. 20009
(202) 483-2600

Florida Division, Inc.
1001 South MacDill Avenue
Tampa, Florida 33609
(813) 253-0541

Georgia Division, Inc.
1422 W. Peachtree Street, N.W.
Atlanta, Georgia 30309
(404) 892-0026

Hawaii Pacific Division, Inc.
Community Services Center Bldg.
200 North Vineyard Boulevard
Honolulu, Hawaii 96817
(808) 531-1662-3-4-5

Idaho Division, Inc.
1609 Abbs Street
P.O. Box 5386
Boise, Idaho 83705
(208) 343-4609

Illinois Division, Inc.
37 South Wabash Avenue
Chicago, Illinois 60603
(312) 372-0472

Indiana Division, Inc.
4755 Kingsway Drive, Suite 100
Indianapolis, Indiana 46205
(317) 257-5326

Iowa Division, Inc.
Highway #18 West
P.O. Box 980
Mason City, Iowa 50401
(515) 423-0712

Kansas Division, Inc.
3003 Van Buren Street
Topeka, Kansas 66611
(913) 267-0131

Kentucky Division, Inc.
Medical Arts Bldg.
1169 Eastern Parkway
Louisville, Kentucky 40217
(502) 459-1867

Louisiana Division, Inc.
Masonic Temple Bldg., 7th Floor
333 St. Charles Avenue
New Orleans, Louisiana 70130
(504) 523-2029

Maine Division, Inc.
Federal and Green Streets
Brunswick, Maine 04011
(207) 729-3339

Maryland Division, Inc.
200 East Joppa Road
Towson, Maryland 21204
(301) 828-8890

Massachusetts Division, Inc.
247 Commonwealth Avenue
Boston, Massachusetts 02116
(617) 267-2650

Michigan Division, Inc.
1205 East Saginaw Street
Lansing, Michigan 48906
(517) 371-2920

Minnesota Division, Inc.
3316 West 66th Street
Minneapolis, Minnesota 55435
(612) 925-2772

Mississippi Division, Inc.
345 North Mart Plaza
Jackson, Mississippi 39206
(601) 362-8874

Missouri Division, Inc.
3322 American Avenue
P.O. Box 1066
Jefferson City, Missouri 65102
(314) 893-4800

Montana Division, Inc.
2820 First Avenue South
Billings, Montana 59101
(406) 252-7111

Nebraska Division, Inc.
8502 West Center Road
Omaha, Nebraska 68124
(402) 393-5800

Nevada Division, Inc.
1325 East Harmon
Las Vegas, Nevada 89109
(702) 798-6877

New Hampshire Division, Inc.
686 Mast Road
Manchester, New Hampshire
03102
(603) 669-3270

New Jersey Division, Inc.
CN2201, 2600 Route 1
North Brunswick, New Jersey
08902
(201) 297-8000

New Mexico Division, Inc.
5800 Lomas Blvd., N.E.
Albuquerque, New Mexico 87110
(505) 262-2336

New York State Division, Inc.
6725 Lyons Street, P.O. Box 7
East Syracuse, New York 13057
(315) 437-7025

Long Island Division, Inc.
535 Broad Hollow Road
(Route 110)
Melville, New York 11747
(516) 420-1111

New York City Division, Inc.
19 West 56th Street
New York, New York 10019
(212) 586-8700

Queens Division, Inc.
111-15 Queens Boulevard
Forest Hills, New York 11375
(212) 263-2224

Westchester Division, Inc.
901 North Broadway
White Plains, New York 10603
(914) 949-4800

North Carolina Division, Inc.
222 North Person Street
P.O. Box 27624
Raleigh, North Carolina 27611
(919) 834-8463

North Dakota Division, Inc.
Hotel Graver Annex Bldg.
115 Roberts Street
P.O. Box 426
Fargo, North Dakota 58102
(701) 232-1385

Ohio Division, Inc.
1375 Euclid Avenue
Suite 312
Cleveland, Ohio 44115
(216) 771-6700

Oklahoma Division, Inc.
3800 North Cromwell
Oklahoma City, Oklahoma 73112
(405) 946-5000

Oregon Division, Inc.
0330 S.W. Curry
Portland, Oregon 97201
(503) 295-6422

Pennsylvania Division, Inc.
Route 422 & Sipe Avenue
P.O. Box 416
Hershey, Pennsylvania 17033
(717) 533-6144

Philadelphia Division, Inc.
21 South 12th Street
Philadelphia, Pennsylvania
19107
(215) 665-2900

Puerto Rico Division, Inc.
(Avenue Domenech 273
Hato Rey, P.R.)
GPO Box 6004
San Juan, Puerto Rico 00936
(809) 764-2295

Rhode Island Division, Inc.
345 Blackstone Blvd.
Providence, Rhode Island 02906
(401) 831-6970

South Carolina Division, Inc.
2442 Devine Street
Columbia, South Carolina 29205
(803) 256-0245

South Dakota Division, Inc.
1025 North Minnesota Avenue
Hillcrest Plaza
Sioux Falls, South Dakota 57104
(605) 336-0897

Tennessee Division, Inc.
713 Melpark Drive
Nashville, Tennessee 37204
(615) 383-1710

Texas Division, Inc.
3834 Spicewood Springs Road
P.O. Box 9863
Austin, Texas 78766
(512) 345-4560

Utah Division, Inc.
610 East South Temple
Salt Lake City, Utah 84102
(801) 322-0431

Vermont Division, Inc.
13 Loomis Street, Drawer C
Montpelier, Vermont 05602
(802) 223-2348

Virginia Division, Inc.
3218 West Cary Street
P.O. Box 7288
Richmond, Virginia 23221
(804) 359-0208

Washington Division, Inc.
2120 First Avenue North
Seattle, Washington 98109
(206) 283-1152

West Virginia Division, Inc.
Suite 100
240 Capitol Street
Charleston, West Virginia 25301
(304) 344-3611

Wisconsin Division, Inc.
615 North Sherman Avenue
P.O. Box 8370
Madison, Wisconsin 53708
(608) 249-0487

Milwaukee Division, Inc.
11401 West Watertown Plank Road
Wauwatosa, Wisconsin 53226
(414) 453-4500

Wyoming Division, Inc.
Indian Hills Center
506 Shoshoni
Cheyenne, Wyoming 82009
(307) 638-3331

In the United States, local units of the American Cancer Society can put you in touch with patient programmes.

United States Cancer Information Service of the National Cancer Institute. Toll free calls may be made from anywhere in the United States. Questions about cancer answered in understandable lay language and latest information provided on treatment and on what resources are available in your region. Almost thirty states have regional toll free numbers. Calls from the others are handled by the Cancer Information Service Office at the National Cancer Institute, 800-638-6694.

National Cancer Institute
National Institutes of Health
Bethesda, Maryland 20014

The Palliative Care Foundation of Canada
288 Bloor St. West
Toronto, Ontario
M5S 1V8
Telephone (416) 922-1281

United States National Hospice Organization
765 Prospect Street
New Haven, Connecticut 06511

Reach to Recovery, a service for women who have had mastectomies, is available in most areas of the United States. Contact the local branch of the American Cancer Society.

Mastectomy Visiting Service in Canada. Consult the nearest branch of the Canadian Cancer Society.

United Ostomy Association
2001 West Beverly Boulevard
Los Angeles, California 90057
Telephone (213) 413-5510

Ostomy Toronto (a branch of the United Ostomy Association)
Box 24, Station A
Willowdale, Ontario
M2N 5S7
Telephone (416) 593-1513

There are branches in all Canadian provinces, totalling more than fifty groups. Contact the local branch of the Canadian Cancer Society. In the United States there are some 500 local chapters. Call the local branch of the American Cancer Society for information.

International Association of Laryngectomies
219 East 42nd Street
New York, N.Y. 10017
Telephone (212) 867-3700

This umbrella organization encompasses more than two hundred clubs including Lost Cord clubs and New Voice clubs. Contact the local branch of the Canadian Cancer Society or the American Cancer Society for information.

CanSurmount
Contact your local branch of the Canadian Cancer Society or the American Cancer Society.

I Can Cope
Contact the American Cancer Society for this programme of eight classes for cancer patients and families.

Living with Cancer
Contact the Canadian Cancer Society for information about this program for patients and families.

Candlelighters (for parents of young cancer patients)
123 C Street S.W.
Washington, D.C. 20003
Telephone (202) 483-9100

Canadian liaison:
Mrs. Edwina Eddy
Box 778
Bedford, Quebec
J0J 1A0

Leukemia Society of America, Inc.
800 Second Avenue
New York, New York 10017
Telephone (212) 573-8484

There are local chapters in the United States. Consult your local telephone directory or the national office listed above.

Make Today Count (for people with cancer and other life-threatening diseases)
P.O. Box 303
Burlington, Iowa 52601
Telephone (319) 753-6112

Bereaved Families of Ontario ,(for families and parents needing help in coping with the death of a child)
214 Merton St.
Toronto, Ontario
M4S 1A6
Telephone (416) 481-3389